<u>Ageless Odyssey</u>

*Unraveling the Secrets to a
Boundless, Vibrant Life*

Jordan A. Sterling

Contents

Introduction

The passage of time is an immutable force, a universal constant that ceaselessly ticks away the seconds of our lives. Despite the inevitability of aging, the human spirit has long been captivated by the tantalizing promise of youth, vitality, and longevity. For centuries, we have been obsessed with uncovering the secrets to staving off the ravages of time and preserving our health, beauty, and vigor as we navigate the complexities of our existence.

In our quest for eternal youth, we have looked to mythology, folklore, and legend for answers, seeking out elusive fountains of youth and magical elixirs. But as we stand on the precipice of unprecedented scientific and technological advancements, it is clear that the true fountain of youth lies within each of us, waiting to be tapped and harnessed.

Welcome to "The Ageless Odyssey: A Comprehensive Guide to Embracing Longevity and Aging Gracefully." This book is designed to be your roadmap to a life of optimal health, vitality, and fulfillment, regardless of the number of candles on your birthday cake. Our journey will take us deep into the fascinating realms of biology, psychology, lifestyle, and technology, as we uncover the secrets to unlocking our full potential for long, vibrant, and meaningful lives.

As you explore the chapters of this book, you will discover that the path to agelessness is multifaceted, encompassing the physical, mental, emotional, and spiritual dimensions of our existence. From the molecular mechanisms of cellular aging to the role of diet, exercise, and mindfulness in promoting optimal well-being, we will delve into cutting-edge research and time-honored wisdom to provide you with a comprehensive understanding of the many factors that influence our experience of aging.

In this journey, we will also address the importance of mental health, resilience, and social connections, recognizing that a fulfilling life is not solely defined by physical health, but also by the richness of our relationships, the depth of our personal growth, and the impact we leave on the world around us.

As we embrace the art of aging gracefully, we will explore the aesthetics of self-care, personal style, and self-expression, acknowledging the power of looking and feeling our best as we traverse the stages of life. We will also delve into the practical aspects of financial planning and legal considerations, providing you with the tools and strategies to secure a future of peace, stability, and fulfillment.

As we look to the future, we will examine the exciting innovations and discoveries on the horizon, from wearable technologies and virtual reality to robotics and personalized genomics, offering a glimpse into the possibilities that await us as we continue to push the boundaries of what it means to age gracefully.

Finally, this book will provide you with a roadmap for integrating these longevity strategies into your daily life, fostering a resilient mindset, nurturing meaningful connections, and embracing the ongoing journey of self-discovery and personal growth that defines the ageless odyssey.

So, take a deep breath, and prepare to embark on a transformative adventure that transcends the boundaries of time and age, as we journey together toward a life of boundless potential, radiant vitality, and unwavering passion. The ageless odyssey awaits, and the fountain of youth within is ready to be unlocked.

Chapter 1: The Fountain of Youth Within

1.1: Uncovering the Mysteries of Aging

1.1.1 - The biology of aging: cellular mechanisms and key players

Aging is a natural and inevitable process that occurs in all living organisms. Despite the fact that it is a universal phenomenon, the exact mechanisms that drive the aging process are still not fully understood. In this chapter, we will delve into the biology of aging, exploring the cellular mechanisms and key players involved in this complex process.

1.1.1.1 Telomeres and Telomerase

One of the key cellular mechanisms involved in aging is the shortening of telomeres, the protective caps on the ends of chromosomes. As cells divide, telomeres gradually become shorter, which ultimately leads to cell senescence and apoptosis. However, some cells, such as stem cells, have the ability to produce telomerase, an enzyme that can extend the length of telomeres and promote cell proliferation. We will explore the role of telomeres and telomerase in the aging process and their potential as targets for anti-aging therapies.

1.1.1.2 DNA Damage and Repair

Another cellular mechanism involved in aging is the accumulation of DNA damage and the gradual decline in the body's ability to repair that damage. We will discuss the sources of DNA damage, such as oxidative stress and environmental toxins, and the various DNA repair mechanisms that operate in cells. We will also examine how this damage and repair process relates to aging and age-related diseases.

1.1.1.3 Mitochondria and Oxidative Stress

Mitochondria are the energy-producing organelles in cells and play a critical role in regulating cellular metabolism. However, mitochondria can also produce reactive oxygen species (ROS), which can cause oxidative damage to cells. Over time, this damage can accumulate and contribute to aging. We will explore the mechanisms of mitochondrial dysfunction and oxidative stress, and their impact on the aging process.

1.1.1.4 Cellular Senescence

Cellular senescence is a state of irreversible growth arrest that occurs in cells as a response to various stressors, such as DNA damage or telomere shortening. Senescent cells can secrete a range of molecules that can have both beneficial and detrimental effects on surrounding tissues. We will discuss the role of cellular senescence in aging and age-related diseases, and the potential of senolytic therapies to target senescent cells and improve healthspan.

1.1.1.5 Epigenetic Changes

Epigenetic changes, which involve modifications to DNA and histone proteins that can affect gene expression, have been implicated in aging and age-related diseases. We will explore the role of epigenetic changes in aging, and the potential of epigenetic therapies to reverse age-related changes in gene expression.

1.1.1.6 Inflammation and the Immune System

Chronic inflammation is a hallmark of aging, and the immune system plays a critical role in regulating this process. We will discuss the various types of immune cells involved in inflammation, and how they can both promote and protect against age-related diseases. We will also examine the potential of immune-modulating therapies to target age-related inflammation.

Conclusion:

In this chapter, we have explored the cellular mechanisms and key players involved in the aging process. Understanding these complex processes is critical for developing effective anti-aging therapies that can promote healthspan and increase longevity. We hope that this chapter has provided valuable insights into the biology of aging and its potential as a target for intervention.

1.1.2 - The role of genetics and epigenetics in the aging process

Aging is a complex process influenced by both genetic and environmental factors. While genetics can play a role in determining lifespan and susceptibility to certain age-related diseases, the interaction between genes and the environment is also crucial in shaping the aging process. In this chapter, we will delve into the role of genetics and epigenetics in aging, exploring the ways in which our genes and epigenetic modifications can impact the aging process.

1.1.2.1 Longevity Genes

Several genes have been identified that are associated with increased lifespan and reduced risk of age-related diseases. These genes include SIRT1, FOXO3, and APOE, among others. We will explore the role of these longevity genes in the aging process, and the potential of gene therapy and gene editing technologies to modulate gene expression and improve health span.

1.1.2.2 Aging and Telomeres

Telomeres, the protective caps on the ends of chromosomes, have been linked to both aging and cancer. Certain genetic variations can influence telomere length and maintenance, and impact the aging process. We will discuss the genetics of telomere biology and their role in aging and age-related diseases.

1.1.2.3 Inherited Risk for Age-Related Diseases

Many age-related diseases, such as Alzheimer's disease and cardiovascular disease, have a genetic component. Certain genetic variations can increase an individual's risk for these diseases, and may also impact the age of onset. We will explore the genetics of common age-related diseases, and the potential for genetic testing and personalized medicine to improve disease prevention and treatment.

1.1.2.4 Epigenetic Changes with Age

Epigenetic modifications, such as DNA methylation and histone modifications, can impact gene expression and contribute to the aging process. We will explore the changes in epigenetic patterns that occur with age, and the potential for epigenetic therapies to modulate gene expression and improve healthspan.

1.1.2.5 Epigenetics and Environment

Environmental factors, such as diet, exercise, and stress, can impact epigenetic modifications and influence the aging process. We will discuss the interaction between epigenetics and environment, and the potential for lifestyle modifications to impact epigenetic patterns and promote healthy aging.

1.1.2.6 Epigenetic Therapies for Aging

Several epigenetic therapies, such as histone deacetylase inhibitors and DNA methyltransferase inhibitors, have shown promise in modulating epigenetic patterns and improving healthspan in animal models. We will explore the potential of epigenetic therapies for human aging, and the challenges and ethical considerations surrounding these approaches.

Conclusion:

In this chapter, we have explored the role of genetics and epigenetics in the aging process. Understanding the complex interplay between our genes, environment, and epigenetic modifications is critical for developing effective anti-aging therapies that can promote healthspan and increase longevity. We hope that this chapter has provided valuable insights into the genetics and epigenetics of aging, and their potential as targets for intervention.

1.1.3 - The impact of lifestyle factors on biological age vs. chronological age

As we age, our chronological age may not always reflect our biological age, which refers to the age of our cells and bodily systems. The impact of lifestyle factors on our biological age is a growing area of research, as we seek to identify ways to promote healthy aging and improve healthspan. In this chapter, we will explore the impact of lifestyle factors on biological age versus chronological age, and the potential for lifestyle modifications to promote healthy aging.

1.1.3.1 The Importance of a Healthy Diet

Dietary choices can have a significant impact on our biological age. We will explore the impact of key nutrients, such as antioxidants and omega-3 fatty acids, on cellular aging and age-related diseases. We will also discuss the potential of dietary interventions, such as calorie restriction and intermittent fasting, to promote healthy aging and improve healthspan.

1.1.3.2 The Benefits of a Plant-Based Diet

Plant-based diets have been linked to reduced risk of age-related diseases and increased longevity. We will discuss the potential mechanisms behind these benefits, and the importance of a varied and balanced plant-based diet for healthy aging.

1.1.3.3 The Role of Supplements

Nutritional supplements, such as vitamins and minerals, have been touted for their potential to promote healthy aging. We will explore the evidence behind these claims, and the potential risks and benefits of supplement use.

1.1.3.4 The Importance of Physical Activity

Regular exercise has been linked to improved healthspan and reduced risk of age-related diseases. We will explore the potential mechanisms behind these benefits, and the importance of a varied and balanced exercise routine for healthy aging.

1.1.3.5 The Role of Strength Training

Strength training has been shown to promote muscle mass, bone density, and metabolic health, all of which can contribute to healthy aging. We will discuss the benefits of strength training for older adults, and the importance of proper form and safety.

1.1.3.6 The Benefits of Aerobic Exercise

Aerobic exercise, such as walking, swimming, and cycling, has been linked to improved cardiovascular health and cognitive function. We will explore the potential mechanisms behind these benefits, and the importance of incorporating aerobic exercise into a balanced exercise routine.

1.1.3.7 The Impact of Chronic Stress

Chronic stress can have a significant impact on our biological age, contributing to cellular aging and age-related diseases. We will explore the potential mechanisms behind this impact, and the importance of stress management techniques for healthy aging.

1.1.3.8 The Benefits of Mind-Body Practices

Mind-body practices, such as meditation, yoga, and tai chi, have been shown to reduce stress and promote relaxation. We will discuss the potential mechanisms behind these benefits, and the importance of incorporating mind-body practices into a healthy lifestyle.

1.1.3.9 The Role of Social Support

Social support has been linked to improved healthspan and reduced risk of age-related diseases. We will explore the potential mechanisms behind these benefits, and the importance of cultivating meaningful relationships for healthy aging.

Conclusion:

In this chapter, we have explored the impact of lifestyle factors on biological age versus chronological age. Nutrition, exercise, stress, and social support are all key factors that can impact our biological age, and promote healthy aging. By making mindful choices and incorporating healthy habits into our daily routines, we can increase our healthspan and enjoy a vibrant, active life as we age.

1.1.4 - The Latest Breakthroughs in Aging Research and Their Potential Implications

Aging is a complex biological process that involves multiple systems and processes in the body. Over the years, there have been significant breakthroughs in aging research that have led to a better understanding of the mechanisms underlying the aging process. In this chapter, we will explore some of the latest breakthroughs in aging research and their potential implications for the field of aging and longevity.

1. Senolytics

Senolytics are a class of drugs that target senescent cells, which are cells that have stopped dividing and are no longer functioning properly. Senescent cells are thought to play a key role in the aging process, as they can release harmful molecules that can damage surrounding tissue and contribute to age-related diseases.

Several studies have shown that senolytics can improve healthspan and lifespan in animal models. In one study, mice treated with a senolytic drug lived 36% longer than control mice. In another study, senolytics were shown to improve cardiovascular function, reduce inflammation, and increase physical function in old mice.

While senolytics are still in the early stages of development, they hold great promise for the treatment of age-related diseases and the promotion of healthy aging.

2. Epigenetic Clocks

Epigenetic clocks are a way of measuring biological age, which is the age of a person's cells as opposed to their chronological age. They work by measuring changes in DNA methylation patterns, which are modifications to the DNA molecule that can affect gene expression.

Recent studies have shown that epigenetic clocks can be used to predict the onset of age-related diseases, such as Alzheimer's disease, and to identify individuals who are at higher risk of developing these diseases. Epigenetic clocks can also be used to track the effectiveness of anti-aging interventions, such as dietary changes and exercise.

3. Mitochondrial Replacement Therapy

Mitochondria are the powerhouse of the cell, producing energy in the form of ATP. However, as we age, the function of our mitochondria declines, leading to a decrease in energy production and an increase in oxidative stress.

Mitochondrial replacement therapy (MRT) is a technique that involves replacing faulty mitochondria with healthy ones. This can be done through a process called mitochondrial transfer, which involves transferring the nucleus of a healthy egg cell to an egg cell with faulty mitochondria.

While MRT is still in the early stages of development, it holds great promise for the treatment of age-related diseases that are caused by mitochondrial dysfunction, such as Parkinson's disease and Alzheimer's disease.

4. Caloric Restriction Mimetics

Caloric restriction is a well-known anti-aging intervention that involves reducing calorie intake while maintaining adequate nutrition. However, caloric restriction is difficult to maintain and may not be practical for everyone.

Caloric restriction mimetics are compounds that mimic the effects of caloric restriction without the need for calorie restriction. They work by activating the same pathways in the body that are activated by caloric restriction, such as the sirtuin pathway and the AMPK pathway.

Several caloric restriction mimetics, such as resveratrol and metformin, have been shown to improve health span and lifespan in animal models. While more research is needed to determine their effectiveness in humans, caloric restriction mimetics hold great promise for the prevention and treatment of age-related diseases.

Conclusion

The latest breakthroughs in aging research hold great promise for the field of aging and longevity. Senolytics, epigenetic clocks, mitochondrial replacement therapy, and caloric restriction mimetics are just a few of the many interventions that are being developed to promote healthy aging and extend lifespan. While more research is needed to determine their effectiveness in humans, these breakthroughs provide hope for

1.2: The Cellular Battlefield

1.2.1 - The process of cellular senescence and its role in aging

Cellular senescence is a complex biological process that occurs when cells stop dividing and lose their ability to function normally. It plays a critical role in the aging process, as senescent cells accumulate in our tissues and contribute to age-related diseases and impairments.

At a cellular level, senescence is triggered by a variety of factors, including damage to DNA, oxidative stress, and inflammation. When a cell reaches a certain point of damage, it undergoes a series of molecular changes that lead to its permanent withdrawal from the cell cycle. This process is known as replicative senescence, and it is characterized by the activation of specific signaling pathways that induce cell cycle arrest and trigger the secretion of a variety of molecules, including cytokines, chemokines, and growth factors.

Senescent cells can have both positive and negative effects on the body. On one hand, they help to prevent the growth of damaged or cancerous cells, and they can also play a role in tissue repair and regeneration. However, when senescent cells accumulate in our tissues, they can cause inflammation, disrupt tissue function, and contribute to a range of age-related diseases, including cancer, cardiovascular disease, and neurodegeneration.

Recent breakthroughs in aging research have focused on the development of drugs and therapies that target senescent cells and remove them from the body. These interventions, known as senolytics, have shown promise in animal studies, and there is growing interest in testing them in human clinical trials.

In addition to pharmacological interventions, lifestyle factors can also play a role in modulating cellular senescence. Regular exercise, a healthy diet, and stress reduction techniques have all been shown to have positive effects on cellular function and may help to reduce the accumulation of senescent cells in the body.

Overall, understanding the process of cellular senescence and its role in aging is a critical area of research with significant implications for human health and longevity. Ongoing studies and new discoveries in this field offer hope for developing effective interventions to prevent age-related diseases and promote healthy aging.

1.2.2 - Antioxidants and free radicals: the battle within our cells

Antioxidants and free radicals are two opposing forces within our cells that play a crucial role in the aging process. Antioxidants are molecules that can neutralize free radicals, which are highly reactive molecules that can damage our cells, including DNA, proteins, and lipids.

Free radicals can be generated in our cells through a variety of processes, including metabolism, environmental toxins, and radiation. When free radicals are left unchecked, they can cause oxidative stress, which can lead to cellular damage and dysfunction.

Fortunately, our bodies have natural defense mechanisms against oxidative stress, including enzymes that can neutralize free radicals, and antioxidant molecules that can scavenge them. Some examples of antioxidants include vitamin C, vitamin E, beta-carotene, and selenium.

Research has shown that a diet rich in antioxidants, such as fruits, vegetables, nuts, and seeds, can help to protect our cells against oxidative stress and reduce the risk of age-related diseases such as cancer, cardiovascular disease, and neurodegenerative diseases.

However, it's important to note that while antioxidants can play a protective role in our cells, too much of a good thing can sometimes be harmful. In some cases, high doses of antioxidant supplements can actually have pro-oxidant effects, potentially promoting oxidative stress instead of reducing it.

Overall, maintaining a healthy balance of antioxidants and free radicals in our cells is key to promoting optimal cellular function and healthy aging. A balanced diet rich in antioxidants, along with regular exercise and stress management techniques, can help to support this delicate balance and promote longevity.

1.2.3 - Strategies to promote cellular repair and regeneration

Cellular repair and regeneration are crucial processes for maintaining healthy and youthful cells in our bodies. As we age, our bodies become less efficient at repairing and replacing damaged cells, leading to various signs of aging and age-related diseases. However, there are several strategies that we can adopt to promote cellular repair and regeneration.

1. Exercise: Regular physical activity is one of the most effective ways to promote cellular repair and regeneration. Exercise stimulates the production of growth factors, which can help repair damaged tissues and promote the growth of new cells. In particular, strength training has been shown to increase muscle mass and improve the function of mitochondria, the energy-producing organelles in our cells.

2. Nutrition: Our diet plays a critical role in promoting cellular repair and regeneration. Consuming a diet rich in antioxidant-rich foods can help neutralize free radicals, which can cause cellular damage. Additionally, consuming sufficient amounts of protein, vitamins, and minerals can support the growth and repair of cells.

3. Sleep: Adequate sleep is crucial for cellular repair and regeneration. During sleep, our bodies produce growth hormone, which plays a vital role in repairing damaged tissues and promoting the growth of new cells. Additionally, sleep deprivation has been linked to increased inflammation, which can impair cellular repair and regeneration.

4. Stress management: Chronic stress can cause cellular damage and impair the body's ability to repair and regenerate cells. Adopting stress management techniques such as

meditation, yoga, or deep breathing can help reduce stress and promote cellular repair and regeneration.

5. Supplements: Certain supplements have been shown to promote cellular repair and regeneration. For example, resveratrol, a compound found in grapes and red wine, has been shown to activate genes involved in cellular repair and longevity. Similarly, omega-3 fatty acids found in fish oil can reduce inflammation and support cellular health.

By adopting these strategies, we can promote cellular repair and regeneration, leading to healthier and more youthful cells, and potentially delaying the onset of age-related diseases. It is important to consult with a healthcare professional before making any significant changes to your lifestyle or incorporating supplements into your routine.

1.2.4 - The emerging field of regenerative medicine and its potential

Regenerative medicine is an exciting new field that holds great potential for treating a wide range of diseases and injuries. At its core, regenerative medicine is based on the idea that the body has an innate ability to repair and regenerate itself, and that this ability can be harnessed to create new treatments for a variety of conditions.

One of the most promising areas of regenerative medicine is stem cell therapy. Stem cells are unique in that they have the ability to differentiate into different types of cells in the body. This means that they can potentially be used to replace damaged or diseased cells, tissues, and organs.

There are several different types of stem cells that can be used in regenerative medicine, including embryonic stem cells, induced pluripotent stem cells, and adult stem cells. Each type of stem cell has its own unique characteristics and potential uses.

Embryonic stem cells, for example, are pluripotent, meaning they have the potential to differentiate into any type of cell in the body. This makes them an incredibly powerful tool for regenerative medicine, but their use is controversial due to ethical concerns related to their origin.

Induced pluripotent stem cells, on the other hand, are created by reprogramming adult cells to revert back to a stem cell state. This eliminates the ethical concerns associated with embryonic stem cells, but they have limitations in their potential applications.

Adult stem cells, such as those found in bone marrow, are also being studied for their potential use in regenerative medicine. These cells are more limited in their ability to differentiate into different types of cells, but they have the advantage of being readily available and easier to obtain than embryonic stem cells.

In addition to stem cell therapy, other regenerative medicine approaches include tissue engineering, which involves creating artificial tissues and organs in the lab, and gene therapy, which involves modifying genes to treat or prevent disease.

The potential applications of regenerative medicine are vast and include treating diseases such as diabetes, heart disease, and Parkinson's disease, as well as injuries such as spinal cord damage and burns. While the field is still relatively new, there have already been several promising clinical trials, and the future of regenerative medicine looks bright.

It is important to note, however, that regenerative medicine is not a magic cure-all, and there are still many challenges that need to be overcome. These include finding ways to control the differentiation of stem cells, ensuring their safety and efficacy, and addressing ethical concerns related to their use. Nonetheless, the potential of regenerative medicine to revolutionize the treatment of disease and injury makes it an exciting field to watch in the coming years.

1.3: Food for Thought: Nutrition and Aging

1.3.1 - The impact of dietary choices on health and aging

Dietary choices play a crucial role in our health and well-being, affecting not only our physical but also our mental health. The food we eat provides us with the necessary nutrients to maintain a healthy body, but it can also contribute to the aging process. In this chapter, we will discuss the impact of dietary choices on health and aging, exploring how different foods and dietary patterns can affect our bodies and potentially influence the aging process.

The Importance of a Healthy Diet

A healthy diet is essential for maintaining optimal health and preventing chronic diseases. A diet rich in fruits, vegetables, whole grains, lean proteins, and healthy fats can help reduce the risk of chronic diseases such as heart disease, diabetes, and cancer. In addition, a healthy diet can also help maintain a healthy weight, which is essential for overall health and longevity.

The Role of Macronutrients

Macronutrients, including carbohydrates, proteins, and fats, are essential for providing the body with energy and supporting various bodily functions. The types and amounts of macronutrients we consume can significantly impact our health and aging. For example, diets high in refined carbohydrates and sugars have been associated with an increased risk of chronic diseases such as diabetes and heart disease. On the other hand, diets high in healthy fats, such as those found in nuts, seeds, and fatty fish, have been shown to have anti-inflammatory effects and may help reduce the risk of chronic diseases.

The Impact of Micronutrients

Micronutrients, including vitamins and minerals, play a crucial role in maintaining optimal health and supporting various bodily functions. These nutrients are essential for maintaining healthy skin, hair, and nails, supporting the immune system, and promoting overall health and longevity. Deficiencies in certain micronutrients, such as vitamin D and iron, can lead to health problems and potentially accelerate the aging process.

The Benefits of Plant-Based Diets

Plant-based diets, such as vegan and vegetarian diets, have gained popularity in recent years due to their potential health benefits. These diets are typically rich in fruits, vegetables, whole grains, legumes, and nuts, which are all excellent sources of fiber, vitamins, and minerals. Plant-based diets have been associated with a lower risk of chronic diseases such as heart disease and cancer, and some studies suggest that they may also help slow the aging process.

The Dangers of Processed Foods

Processed foods, such as fast food, pre-packaged meals, and snack foods, are often high in calories, unhealthy fats, and added sugars. These foods have been associated with an increased risk of chronic diseases such as diabetes and heart disease and may contribute to the aging process. In contrast, whole foods, such as fruits, vegetables, and whole grains, are typically lower in calories and packed with nutrients that can help support health and longevity.

Conclusion

In conclusion, the food we eat plays a significant role in our health and aging. A healthy diet rich in whole foods and low in processed foods can help reduce the risk of chronic diseases and potentially slow the aging process. By making conscious dietary choices, we can support our overall health and well-being and promote longevity.

1.3.2 - Macronutrients, micronutrients, and their role in cellular function

Our bodies require various nutrients to function properly, and a lack of certain nutrients can lead to various health problems.

The two main categories of nutrients are macronutrients and micronutrients.

Macronutrients are nutrients that are required in large amounts and include carbohydrates, proteins, and fats. Micronutrients are nutrients that are required in smaller amounts and include vitamins and minerals. Both macronutrients and micronutrients play important roles in cellular function and overall health.

Carbohydrates are an important source of energy for the body, and they are broken down into glucose to be used by cells. However, not all carbohydrates are created equal. Simple carbohydrates, such as those found in sugary drinks and candies, are quickly absorbed by the body and can lead to spikes in blood sugar levels. On the other hand, complex carbohydrates, such as those found in whole grains and vegetables, are digested more slowly and provide a steady source of energy.

Proteins are essential for the growth, repair, and maintenance of cells. They are composed of amino acids, which are the building blocks of proteins. The body can produce some amino acids, but others must be obtained from the diet. Sources of protein include meat, fish, eggs, beans, and nuts.

Fats are another important source of energy for the body, but they also play a role in cell function. They are important components of cell membranes and are necessary for the absorption of certain vitamins. However, not all fats are created equal. Saturated fats, which are found in animal products and some processed foods, can raise cholesterol levels and increase the risk of heart disease. On the other hand, unsaturated fats, which are found in nuts, seeds, and fatty fish, can have a positive effect on heart health.

Vitamins and minerals are essential for many cellular functions. For example, vitamin C is important for the production of collagen, a protein that is important for skin health. Calcium is important for bone health, and iron is necessary for the production of red blood cells.

In addition to these individual roles, nutrients also work together in complex ways to support overall health. For example, vitamin D is important for the absorption of calcium, which is necessary for bone health. Similarly, vitamin C can help the body absorb iron.

In conclusion, a balanced diet that includes a variety of macronutrients and micronutrients is essential for cellular function and overall health. While individual nutrients play important roles, it is important to consider the interactions between nutrients and the importance of a balanced diet.

1.3.3 - The benefits of plant-based diets and other longevity-promoting eating patterns

The food we eat plays a significant role in our health and longevity. Studies have shown that plant-based diets and other longevity-promoting eating patterns can have a positive impact on our health and may even help to extend our lifespan. In this chapter, we will explore the benefits of plant-based diets and other eating patterns that are associated with longevity.

1.3.3.1 - What is a plant-based diet?

A plant-based diet is a diet that emphasizes whole plant foods such as fruits, vegetables, whole grains, legumes, nuts, and seeds, while minimizing or eliminating animal products. This type of diet is often associated with a lower risk of chronic diseases such as heart disease, diabetes, and certain types of cancer.

1.3.3.2 - The benefits of plant-based diets

Numerous studies have shown that plant-based diets can have a positive impact on our health and longevity. Here are some of the key benefits:

- Lower risk of chronic diseases: Plant-based diets are associated with a lower risk of chronic diseases such as heart disease, type 2 diabetes, and certain types of cancer. A study published in the Journal of the American Heart Association found that people who followed a plant-based diet had a 16% lower risk of developing cardiovascular disease than those who followed a non-vegetarian diet.

- Lower inflammation: Inflammation is linked to many chronic diseases, and plant-based diets have been shown to reduce inflammation in the body. A study published in the Journal of Nutrition found that people who followed a plant-based diet had lower levels of C-reactive protein, a marker of inflammation in the body, compared to those who followed a typical Western diet.

- Improved gut health: Plant-based diets are rich in fiber, which is important for maintaining a healthy gut microbiome. A healthy gut microbiome is associated with a lower risk of chronic diseases and better overall health.

- Lower environmental impact: Plant-based diets have a lower environmental impact than diets that include a lot of animal products. Animal agriculture is a major contributor to greenhouse gas emissions, deforestation, and water pollution, among other environmental problems.

1.3.3.3 - Other longevity-promoting eating patterns

In addition to plant-based diets, there are other eating patterns that have been associated with longevity. Here are a few examples:

- Mediterranean diet: The Mediterranean diet is a plant-based diet that includes fish, poultry, and dairy in moderation, while limiting red meat and processed foods. It is rich in whole grains, fruits, vegetables, nuts, and olive oil. Studies have shown that the Mediterranean diet is associated with a lower risk of chronic diseases and may even help to extend lifespan.

- Blue Zones diet: The Blue Zones are regions of the world where people live the longest, healthiest lives. The Blue Zones diet is based on the eating patterns of people in these regions, which are characterized by a plant-based diet with small amounts of animal products, as well as regular physical activity and social engagement.

- Caloric restriction: Caloric restriction involves reducing calorie intake while still consuming adequate nutrients. Studies in animals have shown that caloric restriction can extend lifespan, and some studies in humans have shown that it may have health benefits as well. However, caloric restriction is difficult to sustain long-term and should only be done under the guidance of a healthcare professional.

1.3.3.4 - Tips for transitioning to a plant-based diet

If you are interested in transitioning to a plant-based diet, here are a few tips to help you get started:

- Start slowly: You don't have to go completely vegan or vegetarian overnight. Start by incorporating more plant-based foods into your diet and

1.3.4 - The role of supplements and functional foods in promoting optimal health

As we age, our bodies undergo various changes that can affect our overall health and wellbeing. Nutritional deficiencies and imbalances are common issues that arise with age, and they can contribute to chronic diseases and other health problems.

One way to address these issues is through the use of supplements and functional foods. These products can provide essential vitamins, minerals, and other nutrients that may be lacking in our diets or that our bodies may have difficulty absorbing. In this chapter, we will explore the benefits and potential risks of supplements and functional foods, as well as some of the key nutrients that are particularly important for healthy aging.

The Benefits of Supplements

Supplements can be a useful tool for addressing specific nutritional deficiencies or for supporting overall health and wellbeing. Some of the key benefits of supplements include:

1. Improved Nutrient Intake: Supplements can provide essential vitamins, minerals, and other nutrients that may be lacking in our diets. This can help to ensure that we are getting all of the nutrients we need for optimal health.

2. Reduced Risk of Chronic Diseases: Supplements have been shown to reduce the risk of chronic diseases such as cardiovascular disease, osteoporosis, and certain types of cancer.

3. Improved Cognitive Function: Some supplements, such as omega-3 fatty acids and B vitamins, have been shown to improve cognitive function and memory in older adults.

4. Enhanced Immune Function: Certain supplements, such as vitamin C, vitamin D, and zinc, can enhance immune function and help to prevent infections.

The Risks of Supplements

While supplements can provide many benefits, they also come with some potential risks. Some of the key risks associated with supplements include:

1. Interactions with Medications: Some supplements can interact with medications, potentially leading to harmful side effects or reduced effectiveness of the medication.

2. Overdose: Overdosing on certain supplements, such as vitamin A and iron, can cause serious health problems.

3. Quality Control Issues: Supplements are not regulated in the same way as medications, which means that there may be inconsistencies in the quality and purity of the products.

4. False Claims: Some supplements may make false or misleading claims about their benefits or effectiveness, which can be misleading for consumers.

Functional Foods

Functional foods are foods that provide health benefits beyond their basic nutritional value. These foods may contain beneficial compounds such as antioxidants, fiber, and probiotics that can help to support optimal health and wellbeing. Some of the key benefits of functional foods include:

1. Reduced Risk of Chronic Diseases: Many functional foods, such as blueberries, spinach, and salmon, have been shown to reduce the risk of chronic diseases such as cardiovascular disease and cancer.

2. Improved Digestive Health: Functional foods such as yogurt and kefir contain beneficial probiotics that can help to support

digestive health and reduce the risk of certain digestive disorders.

3. Improved Cognitive Function: Some functional foods, such as green tea and dark chocolate, have been shown to improve cognitive function and memory.

4. Improved Mood: Certain functional foods, such as fatty fish and walnuts, contain omega-3 fatty acids that have been shown to improve mood and reduce symptoms of depression.

Conclusion

Supplements and functional foods can be powerful tools for promoting optimal health and wellbeing as we age. However, it is important to be aware of the potential risks and to use these products responsibly. Always consult with a healthcare provider before starting any new supplement regimen, and choose high-quality products from reputable manufacturers to ensure their safety and effectiveness. By incorporating supplements and functional foods into a healthy, balanced diet, we can help to support our bodies as they age and reduce the risk of chronic diseases and other health problems.

1.4: The Power of Movement: Exercise and Longevity

1.4.1 - The Long-Term Benefits of Physical Activity on Health and Longevity

Physical activity is one of the most important things we can do for our health and wellbeing. Engaging in regular physical activity can help us maintain a healthy weight, reduce the risk of chronic diseases such as heart disease and diabetes, and even improve our mental health. But did you know that physical activity can also have a profound impact on our longevity?

Studies have shown that people who engage in regular physical activity have a lower risk of premature death compared to those who are physically inactive. This is because physical activity can help prevent many of the chronic diseases that are associated with premature death, such as heart disease, stroke, and certain types of cancer.

But the benefits of physical activity on longevity go beyond just reducing the risk of chronic diseases. Physical activity has also been shown to have a positive impact on cellular aging. As we age, our cells undergo changes that can lead to cellular dysfunction and eventual cell death. This process is known as cellular senescence, and it is one of the key factors in the aging process.

Studies have shown that physical activity can help slow down the process of cellular senescence, leading to healthier cells and a longer lifespan. In fact, one study found that regular exercise can increase the length of telomeres, which are protective caps on the ends of our chromosomes that help prevent cellular damage.

In addition to the benefits on cellular aging, physical activity can also have a positive impact on the immune system. Regular exercise has been shown to boost immune function, which can help prevent infections and illnesses that can be particularly dangerous for older adults.

So how much physical activity is necessary to reap these benefits? According to the Centers for Disease Control and Prevention, adults should aim for at least 150 minutes of moderate-intensity aerobic activity per week, or 75 minutes of vigorous-intensity aerobic activity per week. Additionally, adults should engage in muscle-strengthening activities on two or more days per week.

It's important to note that physical activity is just one piece of the puzzle when it comes to promoting longevity. It's also important to maintain a healthy diet, manage stress levels, and avoid harmful behaviors such as smoking and excessive alcohol consumption. But when it comes to promoting a longer, healthier life, physical activity is certainly a key factor to consider.

1.4.2 - The importance of diverse and engaging fitness routines

Introduction:

Physical activity is a key component of a healthy lifestyle and has been linked to numerous health benefits, including the prevention of chronic diseases, improved mental health, and increased longevity. However, many people struggle to maintain a consistent exercise routine, often due to boredom or lack of motivation. This is where diverse and engaging fitness routines can play a crucial role in keeping people active and committed to their health goals.

The Benefits of Diverse and Engaging Fitness Routines:

1. Increases Adherence: Engaging in a diverse range of physical activities can prevent boredom and burnout, which are common barriers to consistent exercise. Switching up workouts can help keep people engaged and motivated to continue exercising.

2. Promotes Balanced Development: Engaging in a variety of physical activities can promote a more balanced development of different muscle groups and prevent overuse injuries that can result from repetitive exercise.

3. Improves Overall Fitness: Engaging in a diverse range of physical activities can improve overall fitness by challenging the body in different ways and promoting greater cardiovascular health, muscular endurance, and flexibility.

4. Offers a Sense of Adventure: Trying new physical activities and exploring different forms of exercise can offer a sense of adventure and excitement, which can be a powerful motivator to maintain an exercise routine.

Examples of Diverse and Engaging Fitness Routines:

1. Group Fitness Classes: Group fitness classes such as yoga, Pilates, and dance classes offer a diverse and engaging workout while also providing a sense of community and social support.

2. Outdoor Activities: Outdoor activities such as hiking, biking, and swimming offer a change of scenery and fresh air, while also challenging the body in different ways.

3. Interval Training: Interval training involves alternating periods of high-intensity exercise with periods of rest, which can be a highly effective way to improve cardiovascular health and promote weight loss.

4. Mind-Body Practices: Mind-body practices such as tai chi and yoga offer a low-impact, gentle way to exercise while also promoting stress reduction and relaxation.

Conclusion:

Incorporating diverse and engaging fitness routines can be a highly effective way to promote consistent exercise, prevent burnout and boredom, and improve overall health and fitness. By exploring different forms of exercise and staying open to new experiences, individuals can find a fitness routine that is enjoyable, challenging, and sustainable for the long-term.

1.4.3 - Strength, endurance, and flexibility: finding the perfect balance

When it comes to physical activity, there are many different types of exercises and routines that can benefit the body. Some focus on building strength, others on improving endurance, and still others on increasing flexibility. But which is the best for promoting longevity and overall health?

The truth is, a well-rounded fitness routine should include a balance of all three types of exercise: strength training, cardiovascular exercise, and flexibility training. Each has its own unique benefits for the body and can help combat the effects of aging in different ways.

Strength training, or resistance training, involves using weights or resistance bands to challenge and strengthen the muscles. This type of exercise can help to build and maintain muscle mass, which tends to decline with age. In addition, strength training has been shown to improve bone density, which can help prevent osteoporosis, a common condition among older adults.

Cardiovascular exercise, such as running, cycling, or swimming, helps to improve the health of the heart and lungs, and can also help to reduce the risk of chronic diseases like diabetes, heart disease, and stroke. Regular cardio exercise has been shown to improve cognitive function and memory in older adults, and can even help to prevent age-related cognitive decline.

Flexibility training, such as yoga or stretching exercises, can help to improve range of motion, balance, and posture, which can all decline with age. Maintaining flexibility can also help to reduce the risk of falls, a common cause of injury in older adults.

To reap the most benefits from a fitness routine, it's important to incorporate all three types of exercise into your routine. Aim for at least 30 minutes of moderate-intensity aerobic exercise, such as brisk walking or cycling, most days of the week, and at least two days of strength training exercises that target all major muscle groups. Add in some flexibility exercises, such as yoga or stretching, at least two to three times a week to maintain mobility and reduce the risk of injury.

Overall, a balanced fitness routine that includes strength, cardiovascular, and flexibility training can help to promote longevity and overall health, and can combat the effects of aging on the body.

1.4.4 - Motivation, consistency, and creating a sustainable exercise plan

Staying motivated and consistent with exercise can be challenging, especially as we age. However, developing a sustainable exercise plan can help to maintain and even improve our overall health and longevity.

Firstly, it is important to find activities that are enjoyable and sustainable for the individual. For some, this may be traditional gym workouts, while for others, it could be yoga, swimming, or hiking. Experimenting with different activities can help to find what works best for the individual, keeping them engaged and motivated.

Consistency is key when it comes to exercise, and developing a regular routine can help to build healthy habits. Creating a schedule for exercise can help to ensure that it is prioritized and not neglected. This can include scheduling in exercise sessions, finding a workout buddy for accountability, or even joining a class or group.

Additionally, setting achievable goals can be a great motivator. This could be as simple as aiming for a certain number of workouts per week, increasing the duration or intensity of exercise over time, or signing up for a fitness event or challenge.

It is important to recognize that exercise plans should also be sustainable, taking into account individual lifestyles and schedules. This may mean starting with shorter, more manageable workouts and gradually increasing intensity and duration over time. It is also important to listen to the body and adjust workouts as needed to prevent injury and burnout.

Overall, developing a sustainable exercise plan is essential for maintaining health and longevity. By finding enjoyable activities, creating a consistent routine, setting achievable goals, and prioritizing sustainability, individuals can improve their overall physical and mental wellbeing.

1.5: Holistic Health: A Mind-Body-Spirit Approach

1.5.1 - Integrating body, mind, and spirit for optimal well-being

The concept of optimal well-being is a holistic one that encompasses physical, mental, emotional, and spiritual health. Integrating all these aspects of the self can be challenging, but it is essential for achieving optimal well-being. In this chapter, we will explore various strategies for integrating body, mind, and spirit to achieve optimal well-being.

1. The Mind-Body Connection

The mind and body are not separate entities; they are intricately interconnected. Research has shown that negative emotions such as stress and anxiety can have a detrimental effect on physical health, while positive emotions such as joy and happiness can have a beneficial effect. Therefore, it is important to maintain a healthy mind to promote physical well-being.

2. Meditation

Meditation is a powerful tool for integrating the mind and body. It has been shown to reduce stress and anxiety, improve sleep, and increase feelings of well-being. Regular meditation practice can also enhance cognitive function and emotional regulation.

3. Yoga

Yoga is a physical practice that also incorporates breath work and meditation. It is an effective tool for reducing stress, improving flexibility and balance, and promoting overall physical and mental health.

4. Nutrition

Nutrition is an essential component of optimal well-being. A diet rich in whole foods, fruits, and vegetables can help support physical health, while also promoting emotional and mental well-being.

5. Exercise

Exercise is a critical component of optimal well-being. It promotes physical health, reduces stress and anxiety, and improves cognitive function. Finding an exercise routine that is enjoyable and sustainable is key to making it a regular part of daily life.

6. Mindful Breathing

Breathwork is a simple and effective way to connect the mind and body. Mindful breathing exercises can help reduce stress and anxiety, promote relaxation, and improve overall well-being.

7. Gratitude Practice

Practicing gratitude can help shift focus from negative to positive aspects of life. Gratitude has been shown to improve mental and emotional well-being, reduce stress and anxiety, and promote better sleep.

8. Social Connection

Humans are social creatures, and social connections are essential for optimal well-being. Spending time with loved ones, participating in social activities, and volunteering are all ways to build and maintain social connections.

9. Spiritual Practice

Spiritual practice can provide a sense of purpose and meaning in life. Whether it is through organized religion, personal spiritual practice, or a connection to nature, integrating spirituality into daily life can help promote overall well-being.

In conclusion, integrating body, mind, and spirit is essential for achieving optimal well-being. By incorporating practices such as meditation, yoga, nutrition, exercise, breathwork, gratitude, social connection, and spiritual practice into daily life, one can promote physical, emotional, and mental health. It is important to find a balance that works for individual needs and preferences to create a sustainable and enjoyable routine.

1.5.2 - The benefits of ancient practices, such as yoga, Tai Chi, and Qigong

In recent years, there has been an increased interest in ancient practices that promote physical and mental well-being. Practices such as yoga, Tai Chi, and Qigong have been around for thousands of years and have been found to have numerous benefits for overall health and longevity.

Yoga is a practice that originated in ancient India and involves a series of postures and breathing exercises. Practicing yoga has been shown to improve flexibility, balance, and strength, as well as reduce stress and anxiety. A study published in the International Journal of Yoga found that practicing yoga regularly can lead to improved cardiovascular health and a reduction in oxidative stress, which is a key factor in the aging process.

Tai Chi is a form of martial arts that originated in China and involves slow, gentle movements that flow together. Practicing Tai Chi has been found to improve balance, flexibility, and overall physical function. Additionally, studies have shown that practicing Tai Chi can reduce stress and anxiety and improve cognitive function.

Qigong is a Chinese practice that involves slow, gentle movements, deep breathing, and meditation. Practicing Qigong has been found to improve balance, flexibility, and overall physical function, as well as reduce stress and anxiety. Additionally, Qigong has been found to have a positive effect on immune function and can lead to an increase in natural killer cells, which play a role in fighting disease and infection.

One of the key benefits of these ancient practices is their focus on integrating the body, mind, and spirit. By practicing these exercises, individuals are able to connect with themselves on a deeper level and promote overall well-being. Additionally, these practices are low-impact and accessible to people of all ages and fitness levels.

In conclusion, incorporating ancient practices such as yoga, Tai Chi, and Qigong into a daily routine can have numerous benefits for overall health and longevity. These practices promote physical and mental well-being, and their focus on integrating the body, mind, and spirit makes them a powerful tool for promoting overall well-being.

1.5.3 - The role of complementary and alternative medicine in promoting longevity

The desire to live a long and healthy life has led many people to seek out complementary and alternative medicine (CAM) practices that claim to promote longevity. CAM is a diverse range of healthcare practices, products, and therapies that are not considered part of conventional medicine. Many of these practices have been used for centuries in traditional medicine systems such as Ayurveda, Traditional Chinese Medicine

(TCM), and naturopathic medicine. In recent years, some CAM practices have gained popularity in Western countries and are often used in conjunction with conventional medicine.

The use of CAM in promoting longevity is based on the belief that a person's physical, emotional, and spiritual well-being are interconnected, and that achieving a balance between these elements is essential for overall health and longevity. Many CAM practices aim to reduce stress, promote relaxation, and enhance the body's natural healing mechanisms.

One of the most well-known CAM practices that claim to promote longevity is acupuncture, which originated in China thousands of years ago. Acupuncture involves inserting thin needles into specific points on the body to stimulate the flow of energy, or qi, through the body's meridians. Proponents of acupuncture believe that this can help to balance the body's energy and promote overall health and longevity.

Another popular CAM practice is herbal medicine, which involves using natural plant-based remedies to treat a wide range of health conditions. Many herbs and plants have been used for centuries in traditional medicine systems and are believed to have beneficial properties that can help to promote longevity. For example, ginseng, a root that is commonly used in TCM, is believed to have antioxidant properties that can help to protect against cellular damage and promote longevity.

Other CAM practices that claim to promote longevity include meditation, yoga, and tai chi. These practices aim to promote relaxation, reduce stress, and improve physical and mental well-being. Meditation, for example, has been shown to reduce inflammation in the body, which is a key factor in the aging process.

While some CAM practices have been shown to have potential benefits for promoting longevity, it is important to note that many of these practices have not been extensively studied in clinical trials. Additionally, some CAM practices may not be appropriate for everyone and can have potential side effects or interactions with other medications.

Overall, the role of CAM in promoting longevity is an area of ongoing research and debate. While some CAM practices may offer potential benefits, it is important to approach these practices with caution and to consult with a qualified healthcare practitioner before beginning any new therapy or treatment.

1.5.4 - Creating a personalized holistic health plan for a balanced life

In the pursuit of longevity and optimal health, it is important to create a holistic health plan that takes into account all aspects of your physical, mental, and spiritual well-being. This includes not only dietary and exercise habits, but also stress management techniques, social connections, and spiritual practices.

Creating a personalized holistic health plan can be a journey of self-discovery and self-care. It involves examining your current lifestyle habits and identifying areas for improvement, setting goals for yourself, and taking action to achieve those goals.

Here are some steps you can take to create your own personalized holistic health plan:

1. Assess Your Current Lifestyle Habits: The first step in creating a personalized holistic health plan is to assess your current lifestyle habits. Take an honest look at your diet, exercise routine, stress management techniques, sleep habits, social connections, and spiritual practices. Identify areas where you are doing well and areas where you could use some improvement.

2. Set Goals for Yourself: Once you have identified areas where you could use some improvement, set realistic goals for yourself. Make sure your goals are specific, measurable, and attainable. For example, if you want to improve your diet, you might set a goal to eat at least five servings of fruits and vegetables each day.

3. Take Action to Achieve Your Goals: Once you have set your goals, take action to achieve them. This may involve making small changes to your daily routine, such as adding a morning meditation practice or going for a walk after dinner. It may also involve seeking out support from friends, family, or a health coach.

4. Monitor Your Progress: As you work towards your goals, monitor your progress regularly. Keep track of your successes and challenges, and adjust your plan as needed. Celebrate your successes along the way, and be kind to yourself if you experience setbacks.

5. Stay Committed to Your Plan: Creating a personalized holistic health plan is not a one-time event, but an ongoing process of self-discovery and self-care. Stay committed to your plan, and continue to make adjustments as needed. Remember that small, consistent changes can lead to big results over time.

In conclusion, creating a personalized holistic health plan is an important step towards achieving optimal health and longevity. By assessing your current lifestyle habits, setting realistic goals, taking action to achieve those goals, monitoring your progress, and staying committed to your plan, you can create a balanced and fulfilling life that supports your overall well-being.

Chapter 2: The Resilient Mind: Mental Health and Longevity

2.1.1 - The importance of mental resilience and optimism for longevity

Living a long and healthy life is a desire shared by many. While genetics do play a role in determining the lifespan of an individual, there are several lifestyle choices and factors that can influence longevity. This chapter will focus on the importance of mental resilience and optimism for longevity.

Body:

Mental resilience refers to the ability to cope with stress, adversity, and challenges that life throws our way. It involves a set of cognitive, emotional, and behavioral skills that enable individuals to adapt and overcome difficult situations. Studies have shown that individuals with higher levels of mental resilience tend to have better health outcomes and a longer lifespan.

One way in which mental resilience can influence longevity is through its impact on the immune system. Chronic stress has been linked to a weakened immune system and an increased risk of several health conditions, including cardiovascular disease, cancer, and infectious diseases. On the other hand, individuals with higher levels of mental resilience tend to have stronger immune systems, which may help protect them against these health conditions.

Optimism, or a positive outlook on life, is another important factor that can influence longevity. Studies have shown that individuals who are more optimistic tend to have better health outcomes and a longer lifespan than those who are more pessimistic. This may be due to the fact that optimism is associated with a healthier lifestyle, including regular exercise, a healthy diet, and less smoking and drinking.

Furthermore, optimism has been linked to a reduced risk of chronic diseases, such as cardiovascular disease and diabetes. This may be due to the fact that optimism is associated with lower levels of stress and inflammation in the body, which are key factors in the development of these diseases.

Conclusion:

In conclusion, mental resilience and optimism are two important factors that can influence longevity. While genetics do play a role in determining lifespan, lifestyle choices and factors such as mental resilience and optimism can have a significant impact on health outcomes and lifespan. Developing mental resilience and cultivating an optimistic outlook on life can help individuals lead a longer, healthier life.

2.1.2 - Techniques to develop mental toughness, grit, and a positive outlook

In addition to physical health, mental and emotional well-being play a crucial role in promoting longevity. Mental resilience and optimism can help individuals overcome adversity and lead to a more fulfilling life. This chapter will explore some techniques to develop mental toughness, grit, and a positive outlook.

1. Mindfulness meditation: Mindfulness meditation is a practice that involves focusing on the present moment, without judgment or distraction. Regular practice of mindfulness meditation has been shown to decrease stress, anxiety, and depression, and improve attention and cognitive function. Studies also suggest that mindfulness meditation can increase gray matter in regions of the brain associated with emotion regulation and self-control.

2. Cognitive reframing: Cognitive reframing involves changing the way we think about a situation. It is a technique commonly used in cognitive-behavioral therapy (CBT) to help individuals shift their perspective and develop a more positive outlook. For example, instead of thinking "I'm not good at this," reframing could involve thinking "I'm still learning, and with practice, I will improve."

3. Gratitude journaling: Gratitude journaling involves writing down things for which we are grateful. Studies have found that gratitude journaling can lead to increased positive emotions, improved sleep, and better physical health. It can also help individuals focus on the good in their lives, rather than dwelling on negative experiences.

4. Positive self-talk: Positive self-talk involves replacing negative self-talk with positive statements. For example,

instead of thinking "I'm never going to be able to do this," positive self-talk could involve thinking "I may not be able to do this right now, but with practice and effort, I can improve."

5. Goal-setting: Goal-setting involves setting specific, achievable goals and developing a plan to achieve them. It is a technique commonly used in sports psychology and can be applied to any aspect of life. Setting goals can help individuals focus their efforts and increase their motivation and sense of accomplishment.

6. Social support: Social support involves seeking help and support from others. Having a strong social support network has been linked to improved mental and physical health and increased longevity. It can also help individuals cope with stress and adversity.

In conclusion, developing mental toughness, grit, and a positive outlook can have a significant impact on our overall well-being and longevity. By practicing mindfulness meditation, cognitive reframing, gratitude journaling, positive self-talk, goal-setting, and seeking social support, individuals can enhance their mental and emotional resilience and lead a more fulfilling life.

2.1.3 - The science behind gratitude, affirmations, and visualization

Mental well-being is essential for longevity and a healthy lifestyle. In this chapter, we will explore the science behind gratitude, affirmations, and visualization and how these practices can improve our mental and emotional health.

Gratitude

Gratitude is the practice of being thankful for the good things in our lives. It has been shown to have a positive impact on mental health, including reducing symptoms of depression and anxiety, and improving overall well-being. Practicing gratitude can also enhance social relationships and strengthen connections with others.

Research suggests that practicing gratitude can increase the release of dopamine and serotonin, which are neurotransmitters associated with feelings of happiness and well-being. Gratitude can also activate the brain's reward system, similar to how we feel when we receive a gift or experience pleasure.

One way to practice gratitude is to keep a gratitude journal, where we write down things we are thankful for each day. This practice can help us focus on the positive aspects of our lives and shift our attention away from negative thoughts and feelings.

Affirmations

Affirmations are positive statements that we repeat to ourselves to promote self-belief and positivity. Affirmations can help us overcome negative self-talk and increase our confidence and self-esteem.

Research has shown that affirmations can help reduce stress and anxiety, and improve academic and job performance.

Affirmations can also activate the brain's reward system, similar to the effects of gratitude.

To use affirmations, we can choose a positive statement that resonates with us and repeat it daily, either in our minds or out loud. It's important to choose affirmations that feel authentic and believable to us, rather than ones that feel forced or insincere.

Visualization

Visualization is the practice of creating mental images or scenarios in our minds to promote positive outcomes. Visualization can be used to improve performance in sports, academics, or work, and can also help reduce stress and anxiety.

Research suggests that visualization can activate the same areas of the brain as actual experiences, and can help create neural pathways that support positive behavior and outcomes.

To use visualization, we can imagine ourselves achieving a specific goal or outcome, and create a vivid mental image of what that would look and feel like. We can also use guided visualizations, where we listen to a recorded script that guides us through a visualization exercise.

Conclusion

Gratitude, affirmations, and visualization are powerful tools for improving mental and emotional well-being. By practicing these techniques regularly, we can enhance our sense of positivity, reduce stress and anxiety, and promote overall health and longevity.

2.1.4 - Fostering emotional well-being for a fulfilling life

Emotional well-being is an essential aspect of overall health and longevity. Our emotions and mental states can impact our physical health and contribute to chronic conditions, such as cardiovascular disease and autoimmune disorders. Therefore, it is crucial to prioritize emotional health and learn ways to foster positive emotions and emotional resilience.

One technique to promote emotional well-being is through mindfulness meditation. This practice involves paying attention to the present moment without judgment, allowing individuals to observe their thoughts and emotions without getting caught up in them. Studies have shown that mindfulness meditation can reduce symptoms of anxiety and depression and improve overall emotional well-being.

Another way to foster emotional well-being is through engaging in activities that bring joy and fulfillment. Hobbies, social activities, and volunteering can all provide a sense of purpose and connection to others. Additionally, practicing gratitude and focusing on positive experiences can help shift our perspective and increase feelings of happiness and contentment.

Incorporating stress-reduction techniques such as yoga, deep breathing exercises, and progressive muscle relaxation can also be beneficial for emotional well-being. These practices help activate the relaxation response, which can counteract the negative effects of chronic stress on our physical and emotional health.

Lastly, seeking support from loved ones, a therapist, or a support group can provide a safe space to process emotions and develop coping strategies. By prioritizing emotional well-being and utilizing these techniques, individuals can improve their overall quality of life and promote longevity.

2.2: Mindfulness: The Path to Inner Peace

2.2.1 - The benefits of mindfulness on mental and physical health

Mindfulness is a state of mind in which we are aware of our present moment experiences with an attitude of openness, curiosity, and acceptance. It is a skill that can be developed through regular practice and has been shown to have numerous benefits for mental and physical health.

Research has shown that practicing mindfulness regularly can help reduce stress and anxiety, improve sleep quality, boost immune function, and lower blood pressure. Additionally, mindfulness can improve focus, attention, and cognitive function, making it a useful tool for enhancing productivity and overall well-being.

One of the key benefits of mindfulness is its ability to reduce stress. Chronic stress can have negative effects on both physical and mental health, leading to an increased risk of disease, cognitive decline, and mental health disorders. Mindfulness can help reduce stress by increasing our ability to regulate our emotions and manage our reactions to stressful situations.

Mindfulness can also be used to manage anxiety, which is a common mental health concern. By becoming more aware of our thoughts and feelings, we can learn to identify and challenge negative thought patterns and develop a more balanced and realistic perspective on our experiences.

In addition to its benefits for mental health, mindfulness has been shown to have physical health benefits as well. For example, research has found that mindfulness can improve immune function by reducing inflammation in the body. Mindfulness has also been shown to improve sleep quality, which is important for overall health and well-being.

To practice mindfulness, there are a variety of techniques that can be used, including meditation, deep breathing exercises, and body scans. Meditation involves sitting quietly and focusing on the present moment, often by paying attention to the breath. Deep breathing exercises involve taking slow, deep breaths to help calm the body and mind. Body scans involve focusing on each part of the body and noticing any sensations or feelings.

Overall, incorporating mindfulness into daily life can have numerous benefits for both mental and physical health. By becoming more aware of our experiences and learning to manage our reactions to stress and other challenges, we can develop a greater sense of well-being and improve our overall quality of life.

2.2.2 - The transformative power of meditation and relaxation techniques

Meditation and relaxation techniques have been used for thousands of years in various cultures to improve mental, physical, and spiritual well-being. In recent years, there has been a growing interest in the scientific study of these practices and their potential health benefits. The evidence shows that meditation and relaxation techniques can reduce stress, anxiety, depression, and pain, and improve sleep quality, cognitive function, and overall quality of life.

Meditation is a mental practice that involves focusing attention on a specific object, such as the breath or a mantra, and observing one's thoughts and emotions without judgment. There are many different types of meditation, including mindfulness meditation, loving-kindness meditation, and transcendental meditation, each with its unique approach and benefits.

Relaxation techniques include deep breathing, progressive muscle relaxation, and guided imagery, among others. These techniques aim to promote relaxation by reducing physical tension, slowing down the heart rate, and calming the mind.

The transformative power of meditation and relaxation techniques lies in their ability to induce a state of relaxation and reduce the physiological and psychological effects of stress. Chronic stress has been linked to numerous health problems, including cardiovascular disease, diabetes, and depression. By reducing stress, meditation and relaxation techniques can help prevent or alleviate these conditions.

Moreover, research has shown that these practices can have an impact on the brain's structure and function, improving cognitive performance, memory, and attention. Studies have also found that they can increase gray matter in certain areas of the brain, such as the prefrontal cortex and the hippocampus, which are involved in emotional regulation and memory processing.

Incorporating meditation and relaxation techniques into daily life can be challenging, especially for those who are new to these practices. It is essential to find a style that resonates with the individual and to establish a routine that fits into their daily schedule. There are various resources available, including books, apps, and classes, that can provide guidance and support in starting and maintaining a meditation and relaxation practice.

Overall, the evidence suggests that meditation and relaxation techniques are powerful tools for improving mental and physical health and promoting longevity. By reducing stress, improving cognitive function, and inducing relaxation, these practices can help individuals live a more fulfilling and healthy life.

2.2.3 - The role of present-moment awareness in reducing stress and promoting happiness

In our fast-paced, modern world, it can be challenging to remain present in the moment. Many of us are constantly multitasking, juggling multiple responsibilities, and feeling pulled in many directions at once. However, research has shown that practicing present-moment awareness, also known as mindfulness, can have significant benefits for reducing stress, increasing happiness, and improving overall well-being.

Mindfulness is a practice that involves paying attention to the present moment, without judgment. This can involve focusing on the breath, bodily sensations, or simply observing thoughts and feelings as they arise, without getting caught up in them. By cultivating present-moment awareness, individuals can develop a greater sense of clarity, focus, and calm.

One of the main benefits of mindfulness is that it can reduce stress levels. When we are constantly worrying about the future or ruminating on the past, our bodies can become stuck in a state of fight or flight, which can lead to physical and mental health problems. By practicing mindfulness, individuals can learn to let go of these unhelpful thought patterns and focus on the present moment, which can help to calm the nervous system and reduce stress levels.

In addition to reducing stress, mindfulness has also been shown to increase happiness and well-being. By being fully present in the moment, individuals can develop a greater appreciation for the simple pleasures in life, such as spending time with loved ones, enjoying nature, or savoring a delicious meal. Mindfulness can also help individuals to cultivate a greater sense of compassion and empathy towards themselves and others, which can lead to deeper connections and more fulfilling relationships.

There are many different techniques and practices that individuals can use to cultivate mindfulness, including meditation, yoga, and mindful breathing exercises. It's important to find a practice that works for you and to make it a regular part of your routine in order to experience the full benefits of mindfulness.

In conclusion, present-moment awareness, or mindfulness, is a powerful tool for reducing stress, increasing happiness, and improving overall well-being. By practicing mindfulness on a regular basis, individuals can cultivate a greater sense of calm, focus, and clarity, which can help them to navigate the challenges of modern life with greater ease and resilience.

2.2.4 - Developing a personalized mindfulness practice

In recent years, mindfulness has gained immense popularity as a way to reduce stress, improve focus and concentration, and enhance overall well-being. However, the term "mindfulness" is often misunderstood or used in a superficial way. Mindfulness is not just about relaxation or stress reduction; it is a practice that involves intentional and non-judgmental attention to present-moment experiences, thoughts, and emotions. This chapter will explore how to develop a personalized mindfulness practice that is both effective and sustainable.

1. Understanding Your Motivation

The first step in developing a mindfulness practice is to understand your motivation. Why do you want to practice mindfulness? Is it to reduce stress, improve concentration, cultivate compassion, or enhance well-being? Clarifying your motivation can help you choose the type of practice that is most appropriate for you and stay committed to the practice.

2. Choosing a Practice

There are many different types of mindfulness practices, such as breathing meditation, body scan, loving-kindness meditation, and mindful movement. Each practice has its own benefits and challenges, so it's important to choose a practice that suits your goals, preferences, and lifestyle. For example, if you want to reduce stress, you may find breathing meditation helpful, while if you want to cultivate compassion, you may prefer loving-kindness meditation.

3. Setting Realistic Goals

Mindfulness is a skill that requires practice, patience, and persistence. Setting realistic goals can help you stay motivated and avoid frustration. Start with a small amount of time each day, such as 5-10 minutes, and gradually increase the duration as you feel comfortable. It's better to practice for a short time consistently than to practice for a long time sporadically.

4. Creating a Routine

Consistency is key to developing a mindfulness practice. Creating a routine can help you establish a habit and integrate mindfulness into your daily life. Choose a time and place where you can practice without distractions, and make it a priority in your schedule. You may also find it helpful to practice at the same time every day, such as in the morning or before bedtime.

5. Staying Flexible

While consistency is important, it's also important to stay flexible and adaptable. Life can be unpredictable, and there may be times when it's challenging to maintain a regular practice. Rather than giving up, try to find creative ways to practice mindfulness, such as during a break at work, while commuting, or even while doing household chores.

6. Cultivating Mindfulness in Daily Life

Mindfulness is not just about formal meditation practice; it's also about bringing awareness to everyday activities and interactions. You can cultivate mindfulness by paying attention to your breath, body sensations, emotions, and thoughts throughout the day. You can also practice mindfulness while walking, eating, or having a conversation with someone. The more you integrate mindfulness into your daily life, the more natural and effortless it will become.

7. Seeking Support

Developing a mindfulness practice can be challenging, especially if you're new to the practice or if you're dealing with difficult emotions or thoughts. Seeking support from a teacher, mentor, or mindfulness community can be helpful in staying motivated and gaining insight into the practice. You may also find it helpful to read books, attend workshops, or use apps that provide guidance and support for mindfulness practice.

In conclusion, developing a mindfulness practice requires intention, commitment, and patience. By understanding your motivation, choosing a practice, setting realistic goals, creating a routine, staying flexible, cultivating mindfulness in daily life, and seeking support, you can develop a personalized mindfulness practice that enhances your well-being and enriches your life.

2.3: Brain Fitness: Maintaining Cognitive Health

2.3.1 - The secret to maintaining lifelong cognitive health

As we age, cognitive decline can become a major concern. Many people worry about developing memory problems or even dementia in their later years. However, research has shown that there are steps we can take to maintain lifelong cognitive health.

One of the most important factors in maintaining cognitive health is staying mentally active. Engaging in mentally stimulating activities, such as reading, playing games, or learning new skills, has been shown to help preserve cognitive function. In fact, one study found that people who engaged in mentally stimulating activities throughout their lives had a 32% lower risk of developing dementia compared to those who did not.

Another important factor is staying physically active. Exercise has been shown to not only improve physical health but also cognitive function. Regular exercise has been linked to improved memory, attention, and other cognitive abilities.

Diet can also play a role in cognitive health. Eating a diet rich in fruits, vegetables, whole grains, and lean protein sources has been associated with better cognitive function. In particular, foods rich in antioxidants, such as berries, leafy greens, and nuts, may be especially beneficial for cognitive health.

Sleep is also important for cognitive health. Chronic sleep deprivation has been linked to impaired cognitive function and an increased risk of developing dementia. Aim for 7-9 hours of sleep per night to support optimal cognitive health.

Finally, social connections can also support cognitive health. Maintaining close relationships with friends and family, participating in social activities, and volunteering have all been linked to better cognitive function.

In summary, maintaining lifelong cognitive health involves staying mentally and physically active, eating a healthy diet rich in antioxidants, getting enough sleep, and staying socially connected. By incorporating these strategies into our daily lives, we can support our cognitive health and reduce our risk of cognitive decline in later years.

2.3.2 - Brain-boosting activities and strategies for mental fitness

The brain is a remarkable organ that is responsible for our thoughts, feelings, and behaviors. While it is essential to take care of our physical health, it is equally important to maintain cognitive health as we age. Just as regular exercise keeps our bodies healthy, there are also brain-boosting activities that can keep our minds sharp and agile.

1. Engage in mentally stimulating activities:

Activities that challenge the brain, such as puzzles, crosswords, and Sudoku, have been shown to improve cognitive function and memory. Engaging in new activities like learning a new language, playing a musical instrument, or taking up a new hobby can also stimulate the brain and improve mental fitness.

2. Practice mindfulness and meditation:

Mindfulness and meditation have been found to improve cognitive function and reduce stress. Regular practice of mindfulness and meditation can improve attention, concentration, and overall mental well-being.

3. Get enough sleep:

Adequate sleep is crucial for optimal cognitive function. Lack of sleep can lead to cognitive impairments, memory problems, and mood disturbances. It is recommended to get at least 7-9 hours of sleep per night.

4. Exercise regularly:

Regular exercise not only benefits physical health but also promotes cognitive health. Exercise has been found to improve cognitive function, memory, and reduce the risk of cognitive decline.

5. Eat a healthy diet:

A healthy diet rich in fruits, vegetables, whole grains, and lean proteins is essential for maintaining cognitive health. Foods high in antioxidants, such as berries, leafy greens, and nuts, can protect the brain from oxidative stress and inflammation.

6. Stay socially active:

Social engagement and interaction have been found to promote cognitive health and reduce the risk of cognitive decline. Activities like volunteering, joining a club, or attending social events can provide opportunities for social engagement and interaction.

7. Stay intellectually curious:

Continued learning and education have been found to promote cognitive health and reduce the risk of cognitive decline. Reading books, taking classes, and attending lectures are great ways to stay intellectually curious and keep the brain active.

In conclusion, maintaining cognitive health is just as important as physical health. Engaging in brain-boosting activities, practicing mindfulness and meditation, getting enough sleep, exercising regularly, eating a healthy diet, staying socially active, and staying intellectually curious are all great ways to promote optimal cognitive health and well-being.

2.3.3 - The impact of cognitive stimulation on delaying cognitive decline

As we age, cognitive decline becomes increasingly common. This decline can lead to a range of issues such as memory loss, difficulty in learning new skills and processing new information, and even the development of dementia.

Fortunately, research has shown that there are ways to delay cognitive decline and even improve cognitive function in older adults. One such method is through cognitive stimulation.

Cognitive stimulation refers to activities that challenge and engage the brain, helping to maintain and improve cognitive function. Studies have shown that engaging in cognitive stimulation activities on a regular basis can help to delay the onset of cognitive decline, reduce the risk of developing dementia, and improve overall cognitive function.

There are many different types of cognitive stimulation activities that can be effective in promoting cognitive health. Some examples include:

1. Learning a new language or musical instrument

2. Engaging in puzzles and brain teasers such as crossword puzzles, Sudoku, and jigsaw puzzles

3. Playing strategy-based games such as chess or bridge

4. Participating in educational activities such as attending lectures, seminars, or workshops

5. Engaging in artistic activities such as painting, drawing, or sculpture

6. Reading books or other types of literature

7. Participating in social activities such as group discussions, clubs, or volunteer work

8. Using computer programs or apps designed specifically to promote cognitive function

It's important to note that the effectiveness of cognitive stimulation activities depends on the individual's level of engagement and interest in the activity. Activities that are personally meaningful and enjoyable tend to be more effective than those that are not. Therefore, it's important to find activities that align with your personal interests and passions.

In addition to engaging in cognitive stimulation activities, other lifestyle factors such as regular exercise, healthy eating habits, and social engagement have also been shown to promote cognitive health and delay cognitive decline. In summary, incorporating cognitive stimulation activities into your daily routine and adopting healthy lifestyle habits can help to promote cognitive health and delay cognitive decline as you age.

2.3.4 - The role of sleep, nutrition, and exercise in maintaining cognitive health

As we age, it becomes increasingly important to take care of our cognitive health. The good news is that there are many lifestyle factors that can help promote cognitive health, including getting enough sleep, eating a healthy diet, and exercising regularly.

Sleep is essential for cognitive health, as it allows our brains to rest and recharge. During sleep, our brains consolidate memories and clear out toxins that build up during waking hours. Lack of sleep has been linked to impaired cognitive function, including problems with attention, memory, and decision-making.

In addition to getting enough sleep, what we eat can also play a role in cognitive health. Research has shown that a diet high in fruits, vegetables, whole grains, and healthy fats (such as those found in nuts and fish) is associated with better cognitive function and a reduced risk of cognitive decline.

On the other hand, a diet high in processed foods, saturated fats, and sugar has been linked to impaired cognitive function and an increased risk of cognitive decline. This type of diet can also increase the risk of other health problems, such as obesity, diabetes, and heart disease, which can further impact cognitive health.

Exercise is another important factor in maintaining cognitive health. Research has shown that regular exercise can improve cognitive function, including memory, attention, and processing speed. Exercise may also help protect against cognitive decline and reduce the risk of developing conditions such as dementia and Alzheimer's disease.

The exact mechanisms by which exercise promotes cognitive health are not fully understood, but it is thought to be related to increased blood flow and oxygen to the brain, as well as the release of hormones and growth factors that promote the growth and survival of brain cells.

Overall, taking care of our cognitive health requires a multi-faceted approach, including getting enough sleep, eating a healthy diet, and exercising regularly. By making these lifestyle changes, we can promote cognitive health and reduce the risk of cognitive decline as we age.

2.4: Mental Health and Social Connections

2.4.1 - The importance of strong social ties for mental well-being and longevity

In today's fast-paced world, maintaining strong social connections has become more important than ever. While most people think of social ties as just a way to have fun or pass the time, studies show that they are critical to mental well-being and longevity. Indeed, research has shown that people who have strong social connections are not only happier and healthier, but they also live longer than those who are isolated.

Section 1: The Health Benefits of Strong Social Ties

Strong social connections can have a significant impact on mental health. People who have strong social connections are less likely to suffer from depression, anxiety, and other mental health problems. In fact, studies have shown that people who have strong social connections are less likely to develop mental health problems later in life.

Strong social connections can also have a positive impact on physical health. People who have strong social connections have lower levels of stress hormones, which can reduce the risk of chronic diseases such as heart disease, diabetes, and cancer. They are also less likely to suffer from infections and other health problems, as strong social connections can boost the immune system.

Section 2: The Importance of Maintaining Social Ties

Maintaining strong social ties can be challenging, especially in today's fast-paced world where people are often too busy to keep up with friends and family. However, it is critical to make time for social connections, as they are vital to mental and physical well-being.

There are many ways to maintain strong social connections, including:

1. Regularly contacting friends and family: Even a short phone call or text message can help maintain a strong social connection.

2. Participating in group activities: Joining a club or group can help you meet new people and maintain strong social ties.

3. Volunteering: Volunteering is an excellent way to meet new people and give back to the community.

4. Traveling: Traveling can help you meet new people and experience new cultures, which can strengthen social ties.

5. Using social media: While social media should not replace face-to-face interaction, it can be a useful tool for staying in touch with friends and family.

Section 3: Overcoming Social Isolation

Despite the importance of strong social connections, many people struggle with social isolation. Social isolation can be caused by a variety of factors, including age, disability, illness, and a lack of access to transportation.

Fortunately, there are many ways to overcome social isolation, including:

1. Joining a senior center or community group: These groups provide a safe and welcoming environment for older adults to socialize and engage in activities.

2. Participating in online communities: Online communities provide a way for people to connect with others who share similar interests.

3. Seeking help from a social worker: Social workers can provide resources and support to people who are struggling with social isolation.

4. Getting involved in a hobby: Hobbies provide an excellent opportunity to meet new people and develop social connections.

Conclusion:

In conclusion, strong social connections are critical to mental and physical well-being. While maintaining strong social ties can be challenging, it is essential to make time for them, as they can have a significant impact on health and longevity. By participating in group activities, volunteering, and maintaining regular contact with friends and family, you can strengthen your social connections and improve your overall well-being.

2.4.2 - Strategies for cultivating and maintaining meaningful relationships

Humans are social creatures, and research shows that social connections are essential for our physical and mental health. Strong social ties have been linked to greater happiness, reduced stress, and a longer lifespan. Conversely, social isolation can have negative health consequences, such as increased risk of depression, anxiety, and chronic disease. Therefore, it is crucial to cultivate and maintain meaningful relationships throughout our lives.

Here are some strategies for developing and maintaining strong social connections:

1. Prioritize social relationships: Just as you make time for other important activities like exercise or work, it is crucial to prioritize time for social relationships. Make plans with friends, schedule regular phone or video chats with loved ones who live far away, or join a group or club that interests you.

2. Practice active listening: When spending time with others, practice active listening by giving your full attention to the conversation. Avoid interrupting and ask questions to show your interest and understanding.

3. Express gratitude and appreciation: Regularly expressing gratitude and appreciation towards your loved ones can strengthen your relationships. Show your appreciation by sending a heartfelt note, offering a thoughtful gift, or simply saying thank you.

4. Practice forgiveness: Conflict is inevitable in any relationship. Practicing forgiveness, letting go of grudges, and moving on from conflicts can help strengthen relationships and promote well-being.

5. Embrace vulnerability: Being vulnerable with others can foster deeper connections. Share your thoughts, feelings, and experiences with those you trust, and be open to receiving their support and empathy in return.

6. Seek out new social opportunities: Joining a new group, taking a class, or volunteering can provide opportunities to meet new people and expand your social circle.

7. Nurture long-distance relationships: Maintaining relationships with those who live far away can be challenging but is essential for our well-being. Make an effort to stay in touch regularly through phone calls, video chats, or even sending care packages.

In summary, prioritizing social connections and implementing strategies like active listening, expressing gratitude, forgiveness, vulnerability, seeking out new social opportunities, and nurturing long-distance relationships can help cultivate and maintain meaningful relationships. These relationships play a crucial role in our overall health and well-being, contributing to a fulfilling and satisfying life.

2.4.3 - The role of altruism and community engagement in promoting mental health

In today's fast-paced and individualistic world, it's easy to feel disconnected and lonely. Social isolation is a growing problem that can have serious consequences on mental health and well-being. However, research has shown that engaging in altruistic behavior and community involvement can have a positive impact on mental health, promoting a sense of purpose and belonging that can lead to greater life satisfaction.

Altruism, or the act of helping others without expecting anything in return, has been linked to increased happiness, lower levels of stress, and a greater sense of meaning and purpose in life. Engaging in acts of kindness, whether small or large, can boost mood and promote positive emotions such as empathy and compassion. Studies have shown that volunteering, in particular, can have significant benefits for mental health. Volunteers often report lower levels of depression, greater life satisfaction, and a greater sense of purpose in life. In addition, volunteering can increase social connections and provide a sense of belonging to a larger community.

Community engagement, or involvement in social and cultural events, can also have a positive impact on mental health. Participating in community events and groups can increase social support and promote a sense of belonging. Research has shown that a strong social network can protect against mental health problems and increase resilience in the face of stress.

There are many ways to get involved in altruistic behavior and community engagement. Volunteering at a local charity, participating in a community event or festival, or joining a social club are just a few examples. The key is to find activities that align with personal interests and values. By engaging in activities that feel meaningful and purposeful, individuals can experience the benefits of altruism and community involvement while also enhancing their mental health and well-being.

In conclusion, promoting mental health and well-being requires more than just individual efforts. Community engagement and altruistic behavior can be powerful tools for promoting a sense of purpose, belonging, and connection. By getting involved in activities that align with personal values and interests, individuals can experience the benefits of social connections and contribute to the well-being of others.

2.4.4 - Finding balance between solitude and social interaction

In our modern society, we are constantly bombarded with social media notifications, text messages, and phone calls, making it difficult to find solitude and quiet time. On the other hand, we also know that social interaction is essential for our mental and emotional well-being. So, how do we find balance between solitude and social interaction?

Finding solitude is important for our mental health as it allows us to reflect, recharge, and refocus. Solitude can take many forms, such as meditation, taking a walk alone, or simply disconnecting from technology. In order to find balance, it's important to prioritize and schedule in time for solitude, just as you would with social events or work.

Social interaction, on the other hand, is also crucial for our mental and emotional well-being. Human beings are social creatures, and we thrive on connection with others. Social interaction can take many forms, such as spending time with loved ones, participating in group activities, or even just striking up a conversation with a stranger.

It's important to remember that social interaction doesn't always have to be in person. In today's digital age, we have access to a variety of ways to connect with others, including social media, online forums, and video chats. However, it's important to be intentional with our social interactions and make sure they are meaningful and fulfilling.

Ultimately, finding balance between solitude and social interaction is about being intentional and prioritizing both in our lives. By taking time for ourselves, we can recharge and refocus, which can lead to more meaningful and fulfilling social interactions. And by connecting with others, we can cultivate strong relationships and a sense of community, which is essential for our mental and emotional well-being.

Chapter 3: The Art of Aging Gracefully: Aesthetics and Self-Care

3.1: A Radiant Glow: Skincare and Aging

3.1.1 - The science behind skin aging and its contributing factors

In this chapter, we will explore the science behind skin aging and its contributing factors. As we age, our skin undergoes a series of changes that result in wrinkles, age spots, and a loss of elasticity. These changes are caused by both intrinsic and extrinsic factors.

Intrinsic factors are those that are determined by our genetics and are a natural part of the aging process. As we age, the production of collagen and elastin in our skin decreases, leading to a loss of firmness and elasticity. In addition, our skin becomes thinner and drier, making it more susceptible to damage.

Extrinsic factors, on the other hand, are external factors that can accelerate the aging process. These include UV radiation from the sun, environmental pollution, smoking, and poor nutrition. Exposure to UV radiation is one of the primary extrinsic factors that contribute to skin aging. UV radiation causes damage to the DNA in our skin cells, leading to the formation of wrinkles, age spots, and other signs of aging.

Other extrinsic factors, such as pollution and smoking, can also contribute to skin aging by causing oxidative stress in the skin. Oxidative stress occurs when there is an imbalance between the production of free radicals and the body's ability to neutralize them. This can lead to inflammation, which can accelerate the aging process.

Poor nutrition can also contribute to skin aging by depriving the skin of the nutrients it needs to maintain its health and vitality. For example, a diet that is high in sugar and processed foods can lead to the formation of advanced glycation end-products (AGEs), which can damage collagen and elastin in the skin.

Overall, the aging process is complex and multifactorial. While some factors, such as genetics, are beyond our control, there are many steps we can take to slow down the aging process and keep our skin looking youthful and healthy. In the following chapters, we will explore some of these strategies in more detail.

3.1.2 - Building a comprehensive skincare routine for youthful skin

Beautiful and youthful-looking skin is something that most of us desire. However, as we age, our skin starts to lose its elasticity, firmness, and radiance due to various internal and external factors. These factors include genetics, lifestyle choices, environmental pollution, exposure to sunlight, and improper skincare. But the good news is that we can slow down the aging process and maintain healthy, glowing skin with the right skincare routine. In this chapter, we will discuss the science behind skin aging and the contributing factors. We will also provide comprehensive guidance on building a skincare routine that will help maintain youthful skin.

Science behind Skin Aging:

Skin aging is a complex biological process that is influenced by both intrinsic and extrinsic factors. Intrinsic aging is a natural process that occurs as we age, while extrinsic aging is caused by external factors such as sun exposure, pollution, and lifestyle habits.

One of the main causes of intrinsic aging is a decrease in the production of collagen and elastin, which are essential proteins that provide the skin with its structure, elasticity, and firmness. As we age, the production of these proteins decreases, causing the skin to become thinner, drier, and more prone to wrinkles and sagging.

Extrinsic aging is caused by external factors such as sun exposure, pollution, and lifestyle habits. The sun's harmful UV rays can cause damage to the skin cells, leading to wrinkles, age spots, and dryness. Environmental pollution can also damage the skin by causing inflammation and oxidative stress. Lifestyle habits such as smoking, alcohol consumption, and an unhealthy diet can also accelerate skin aging.

Building a Comprehensive Skincare Routine:

A comprehensive skincare routine should consist of the following steps:

1. Cleansing: Cleansing is the first and most crucial step in any skincare routine. It helps to remove dirt, oil, and impurities from the skin, which can clog pores and lead to breakouts. Choose a gentle, pH-balanced cleanser that suits your skin type.

2. Toning: Toning helps to balance the skin's pH levels and prepare it for the next steps in your routine. Use a toner that contains ingredients such as hyaluronic acid, glycolic acid, or salicylic acid, depending on your skin's needs.

3. Serum: A serum is a concentrated formula that delivers active ingredients deep into the skin. Choose a serum that contains antioxidants such as vitamin C, vitamin E, or retinol, which help to fight free radical damage and promote collagen production.

4. Eye Cream: The skin around the eyes is delicate and prone to wrinkles and fine lines. Use an eye cream that contains ingredients such as caffeine, hyaluronic acid, or retinol, which help to hydrate, firm, and brighten the skin around the eyes.

5. Moisturizer: Moisturizer helps to hydrate the skin and protect it from external factors such as pollution and UV rays. Choose a moisturizer that contains ingredients such as ceramides, hyaluronic acid, or niacinamide, depending on your skin's needs.

6. Sunscreen: Sunscreen is essential to protect the skin from UV damage, which is the primary cause of extrinsic aging. Choose a broad-spectrum sunscreen with an SPF of at least 30 and apply it every day, even on cloudy days.

Conclusion:

A comprehensive skincare routine can help slow down the aging process and maintain youthful-looking skin. Understanding the science behind skin aging and the contributing factors is essential to building an effective skincare routine. By following the steps mentioned above and choosing the right products that suit your skin's needs, you can achieve healthy, radiant, and youthful-looking skin.

3.1.3 - Innovative skincare technologies and treatments

Advancements in science and technology have paved the way for new skincare treatments and technologies that can help combat the signs of aging and promote youthful-looking skin. These innovative treatments have been developed based on extensive research and clinical studies, making them highly effective in improving skin texture, tone, and overall appearance.

Here are some of the most popular and effective innovative skincare technologies and treatments available today:

1. Light Therapy

Light therapy involves the use of different types of light to stimulate the skin's natural healing processes, promote collagen production, and reduce the appearance of fine lines and wrinkles. LED (light-emitting diode) light therapy, in particular, has been shown to be highly effective in improving skin texture and reducing the signs of aging. Red light stimulates collagen production, while blue light helps to reduce acne breakouts.

2. Microcurrent Therapy

Microcurrent therapy uses low-level electrical currents to stimulate facial muscles and improve skin tone and texture. This treatment can help to reduce the appearance of fine lines and wrinkles, improve facial contour, and enhance skin hydration.

3. Radiofrequency (RF) Therapy

RF therapy uses energy waves to stimulate collagen production and improve skin elasticity. This treatment can help to reduce the appearance of fine lines and wrinkles, tighten sagging skin, and improve skin texture and tone.

4. Laser Skin Resurfacing

Laser skin resurfacing involves the use of a laser to remove the outer layers of damaged skin, revealing fresh, new skin underneath. This treatment can help to reduce the appearance of fine lines and wrinkles, improve skin texture and tone, and reduce the appearance of scars and hyperpigmentation.

5. Platelet-Rich Plasma (PRP) Therapy

PRP therapy involves the injection of platelet-rich plasma, a component of your own blood that contains growth factors, into the skin. This treatment can help to improve skin texture and tone, reduce the appearance of fine lines and wrinkles, and enhance overall skin health and vitality.

6. Hyaluronic Acid (HA) Fillers

HA fillers are injectable treatments that use a naturally occurring substance in the body, hyaluronic acid, to add volume to the skin and reduce the appearance of fine lines and wrinkles. This treatment can help to enhance facial contour and restore a more youthful appearance.

7. Chemical Peels

Chemical peels involve the application of a chemical solution to the skin, which helps to remove the outer layers of damaged skin and reveal fresh, new skin underneath. This treatment can help to reduce the appearance of fine lines and wrinkles, improve skin texture and tone, and reduce the appearance of scars and hyperpigmentation.

Overall, these innovative skincare technologies and treatments offer a wide range of benefits for those seeking to improve their skin's health and appearance. It's important to consult with a skincare professional to determine which treatment is best suited for your individual needs and skin type.

3.1.4 - The role of nutrition, hydration, and sleep in maintaining healthy skin

Our skin is the largest organ in the body and plays a crucial role in protecting us from external damage. It is also a reflection of our internal health, and what we eat, drink, and how much rest we get can greatly impact its appearance and overall health.

In this chapter, we will discuss the role of nutrition, hydration, and sleep in maintaining healthy skin. We will explore how our diet affects the skin, the importance of hydration, and how getting enough sleep can help keep our skin looking and feeling healthy.

The Impact of Nutrition on Skin Health

The foods we eat can have a significant impact on the health of our skin. A diet that is high in processed foods, sugar, and unhealthy fats can contribute to skin problems such as acne, wrinkles, and dullness. On the other hand, a diet that is rich in vitamins, minerals, and antioxidants can help improve the appearance and health of our skin.

Vitamins and Minerals

Certain vitamins and minerals are essential for healthy skin. For example, vitamin C plays a key role in collagen synthesis, which is essential for skin elasticity and firmness. Vitamin E is an antioxidant that can help protect the skin from damage caused by free radicals. Zinc is important for wound healing and can help reduce inflammation, which is beneficial for acne-prone skin.

Sources of these essential vitamins and minerals can be found in a variety of foods. Vitamin C can be found in citrus fruits, kiwi, strawberries, and bell peppers. Vitamin E can be found in nuts, seeds, and vegetable oils. Zinc can be found in lean meats, seafood, and whole grains.

Antioxidants

Antioxidants are compounds that help protect the skin from damage caused by free radicals, which are molecules that can damage cells and contribute to aging. Antioxidants can be found in a variety of fruits and vegetables, as well as in some nuts and seeds.

Some of the most potent antioxidant-rich foods include berries, dark leafy greens, and brightly colored fruits and vegetables like tomatoes, sweet potatoes, and blueberries. Including a variety of these antioxidant-rich foods in your diet can help protect your skin from damage and keep it looking healthy and youthful.

Hydration and Skin Health

Staying hydrated is essential for maintaining healthy skin. When we are dehydrated, our skin can become dry, flaky, and dull. Drinking enough water can help keep the skin hydrated and improve its elasticity and texture.

In addition to drinking water, there are other ways to hydrate the skin from the outside in. Using a moisturizer can help keep the skin hydrated, and choosing a moisturizer with ingredients like hyaluronic acid can help attract and retain moisture in the skin.

Sleep and Skin Health

Getting enough sleep is essential for overall health, including the health of our skin. During sleep, our body repairs and regenerates cells, which is important for maintaining healthy skin.

Not getting enough sleep can contribute to a variety of skin problems, including dark circles under the eyes, dullness, and an increase in fine lines and wrinkles. Aim for 7-8 hours of sleep each night to help keep your skin looking and feeling its best.

Conclusion

The health of our skin is closely tied to our overall health and wellbeing. Eating a healthy diet rich in vitamins, minerals, and antioxidants, staying hydrated, and getting enough sleep are all essential for maintaining healthy skin. By making these healthy habits a priority, you can help protect and improve the appearance and health of your skin.

3.2: Hair Care: Maintaining Strength, Shine, and Vitality

3.2.1 - Understanding the biology of hair and its changes with age

Introduction:

Hair is one of the most prominent features of our appearance and is an important aspect of our identity. It protects our scalp from UV rays, cold, and other environmental factors, and provides us with a sense of pride and confidence. However, as we age, our hair goes through changes that can be distressing and affect our self-esteem. It becomes thinner, loses its shine, and starts to fall out. In this chapter, we will explore the biology of hair and its changes with age.

Biology of Hair:

Hair is composed of a protein called keratin that is produced by specialized cells called keratinocytes located in the hair follicles. Hair growth is a cyclical process that goes through three phases: anagen, catagen, and telogen. During the anagen phase, the hair grows actively and can last for several years. In the catagen phase, the hair stops growing and the follicle shrinks. In the telogen phase, the hair falls out and the follicle remains inactive for a few months before the cycle restarts.

Hair Changes with Age:

As we age, the hair growth cycle slows down, and the anagen phase becomes shorter. This results in thinner hair that grows more slowly and is more susceptible to damage. The hair follicles also shrink, which affects the amount and quality of hair produced. The hair strands become less dense, and the hair may become dry, brittle, and less shiny.

In addition to the natural aging process, other factors can also contribute to hair changes. Hormonal changes, such as those that occur during menopause, can affect the hair growth cycle and cause hair thinning. Certain medications, such as chemotherapy drugs, can also affect hair growth and cause hair loss.

Maintaining Healthy Hair:

While it is not possible to prevent all hair changes with age, there are steps you can take to maintain healthy hair. Eating a balanced diet rich in nutrients such as protein, vitamins, and minerals can help promote healthy hair growth. Staying hydrated and getting enough sleep can also help support healthy hair.

Using gentle hair care products and avoiding harsh chemicals or treatments can help minimize damage to the hair. Avoiding excessive heat styling or brushing can also help reduce hair breakage.

Conclusion:

In conclusion, understanding the biology of hair and its changes with age can help us take steps to maintain healthy hair. While some hair changes are a natural part of aging, taking care of our hair can help minimize damage and promote healthy hair growth.

3.2.2 - Tips for maintaining healthy hair throughout your life

Introduction:

The state of your hair is an indication of your overall health and wellbeing. Therefore, taking care of your hair is crucial for maintaining healthy, strong, and shiny locks. However, as we age, our hair undergoes various changes, including thinning, graying, and loss of elasticity. In this chapter, we will explore some of the best tips for maintaining healthy hair throughout your life, regardless of age.

1. Eat a Nutritious Diet:

The foods you eat play a vital role in maintaining healthy hair. A diet rich in vitamins, minerals, and proteins can help promote hair growth and prevent hair loss. Some of the best foods for healthy hair include leafy green vegetables, nuts, fish, eggs, and berries.

2. Avoid Harsh Chemicals:

Harsh chemicals in hair products such as shampoos, conditioners, and hair dyes can damage your hair and scalp. Avoid using products with ingredients such as sulfates, parabens, and phthalates. Opt for natural and organic hair products that are gentle on your hair.

3. Protect Your Hair from the Sun:

The sun's UV rays can cause damage to your hair, making it dry, brittle, and prone to breakage. When going out in the sun, wear a hat or use a scarf to protect your hair from the sun.

4. Massage Your Scalp:

Massaging your scalp can help promote healthy hair growth by improving blood flow to your hair follicles. Use your fingertips to massage your scalp for a few minutes daily.

5. Avoid Heat Styling:

Heat styling tools such as straighteners, curlers, and hairdryers can damage your hair and cause split ends. Avoid using heat styling tools as much as possible. If you must use them, use a heat protectant spray and set the temperature to a lower setting.

6. Stay Hydrated:

Drinking plenty of water can help keep your hair hydrated, soft, and shiny. Aim to drink at least eight glasses of water daily.

7. Get Regular Haircuts:

Regular haircuts can help maintain the health of your hair. Trimming your hair every six to eight weeks can help prevent split ends and breakage, which can lead to hair loss.

Conclusion:

By following these tips, you can maintain healthy, shiny, and strong hair throughout your life. Remember that the health of your hair is a reflection of your overall health and wellbeing, so it's important to take care of your hair from the inside out. A nutritious diet, gentle hair products, protection from the sun, regular scalp massages, avoiding heat styling, staying hydrated, and regular haircuts are all important steps to take for healthy and beautiful hair.

3.2.3 - Addressing common hair concerns: thinning, graying, and damage

Hair is an important aspect of one's appearance and can greatly impact their self-esteem and confidence. As we age, our hair goes through changes, and many people experience concerns such as thinning, graying, and damage. In this chapter, we will discuss these common hair concerns and offer tips for addressing them.

Thinning hair:

Hair thinning is a common concern that affects both men and women. It can be caused by a variety of factors, including genetics, hormonal changes, medication, and nutritional deficiencies. To address thinning hair, it's important to first identify the underlying cause. For example, if the cause is a nutritional deficiency, supplementing with vitamins and minerals like biotin, iron, and zinc may help promote hair growth. For hormonal causes, medication or hormone replacement therapy may be necessary. It's also important to avoid harsh styling practices like tight braids and high-heat styling tools, as these can cause further damage to already weakened hair. Consider using gentle hair products and investing in a silk pillowcase to reduce friction and breakage.

Graying hair:

Graying hair is a natural part of aging and occurs when the hair follicle stops producing pigment. While there's no way to reverse graying hair, there are ways to slow down the process and maintain healthy hair. To prevent premature graying, it's important to maintain a healthy diet rich in vitamins and minerals, avoid smoking, and reduce stress levels. Additionally, using hair products with UV protection can prevent damage from the sun and slow down the graying process.

Damaged hair:

Damage to hair can occur from a variety of factors, including heat styling, chemical treatments, and environmental factors like pollution and harsh weather conditions. To address damaged hair, it's important to first identify the cause and adjust hair care practices accordingly. Consider reducing the use of heat styling tools and using protective products like heat protectant sprays. Deep conditioning treatments can help nourish and repair damaged hair, and regular trims can prevent split ends from worsening. Additionally, wearing a hat or scarf can protect hair from the sun and harsh weather conditions.

In conclusion, addressing common hair concerns like thinning, graying, and damage can greatly improve one's overall hair health and boost confidence. By identifying the underlying cause and adjusting hair care practices accordingly, individuals can promote healthy hair and maintain a youthful appearance.

3.2.4 - The benefits of a holistic approach to hair care

Hair is an important aspect of our appearance, and it plays a significant role in our overall self-esteem and confidence. While there are a plethora of products on the market promising to improve the health and appearance of our hair, taking a holistic approach to hair care can provide a more comprehensive and long-term solution.

A holistic approach to hair care involves considering the entire person, including their lifestyle, diet, and overall health, rather than just focusing on the hair itself. This approach recognizes that hair is an extension of the body and that its health is intertwined with the health of the entire body.

One of the main benefits of a holistic approach to hair care is that it can promote healthier, stronger, and more resilient hair. By focusing on overall health, individuals can address underlying issues such as nutrient deficiencies, hormonal imbalances, and stress that can impact hair health. Eating a well-balanced diet rich in vitamins and minerals such as iron, zinc, and biotin, can help support healthy hair growth, while managing stress through techniques such as meditation and exercise can improve overall hair health.

Another benefit of a holistic approach to hair care is that it can reduce reliance on harmful hair products. Many conventional hair care products contain chemicals such as sulfates, parabens, and synthetic fragrances that can strip the hair of its natural oils, leading to dryness and breakage. By incorporating natural and organic hair care products into their routine, individuals can reduce their exposure to harmful chemicals and promote a healthier, more sustainable hair care routine.

In addition, taking a holistic approach to hair care can also promote a more sustainable and environmentally-friendly approach to hair care. By choosing natural and organic products and reducing reliance on hair styling tools that require electricity, individuals can reduce their carbon footprint and support a more eco-friendly lifestyle.

Overall, a holistic approach to hair care can provide numerous benefits, including promoting healthier hair, reducing reliance on harmful hair products, and supporting a more sustainable lifestyle. By prioritizing overall health and well-being, individuals can achieve not only healthier hair but also a healthier and more fulfilling life.

3.3: Dressing for Success: Fashion and Personal Style

3.3.1 - The psychology of personal style and its impact on self-image and confidence

Personal style is more than just clothing or fashion accessories. It's a reflection of who you are and how you present yourself to the world. In this chapter, we will discuss the psychology of personal style and its impact on self-image and confidence. We will explore how personal style influences our perception of ourselves and others and how it can affect our behavior and emotions.

The Psychology of Personal Style:

Personal style is a complex and multifaceted concept that encompasses not only the clothing we wear but also our grooming, posture, and nonverbal communication. Our personal style is influenced by various factors, including our personality, culture, social status, and personal values. It's also shaped by our experiences, such as our upbringing, education, and relationships.

Research has shown that personal style can have a significant impact on our self-image and confidence. When we feel good about our appearance, we are more likely to feel confident and capable. We may be more assertive in our interactions with others and feel more comfortable taking risks.

Personal style can also affect our emotions. Studies have found that wearing clothing that we associate with positive emotions, such as comfort or joy, can lead to increased feelings of happiness and well-being.

The Role of Self-Expression:

Personal style is an essential tool for self-expression. It allows us to communicate our identity and values to the world around us. When we dress in a way that reflects our personality and interests, we are more likely to feel authentic and genuine. Personal style can also be a form of creative expression, allowing us to experiment with different looks and aesthetics.

Personal Style and Perception:

Our personal style can also influence how others perceive us. Clothing and grooming can send subtle signals about our personality, social status, and cultural background. We may be judged based on our appearance, both positively and negatively.

Research has shown that our personal style can also affect our behavior. For example, dressing professionally may lead to more productive and efficient work behavior, while wearing casual clothing may promote a more relaxed and creative mindset.

Creating a Personal Style:

Developing a personal style that reflects your personality and values takes time and experimentation. It's important to consider factors such as comfort, practicality, and appropriateness for different settings. It's also essential to be open to feedback from others and to be willing to adapt and evolve your style over time.

Conclusion:

Personal style is a powerful tool for self-expression and can have a significant impact on our self-image and confidence. It's a reflection of who we are and how we want to present ourselves to the world. By understanding the psychology of personal style and its influence on our behavior and emotions, we can develop a style that not only looks good but also feels authentic and genuine.

3.3.2 - Dressing for your body shape, age, and lifestyle

The way you dress can have a significant impact on how you feel about yourself and how others perceive you. Dressing well can boost your confidence, enhance your mood, and even improve your performance in certain situations. But how do you choose the right clothes for your body shape, age, and lifestyle?

In this chapter, we will discuss some practical tips to help you dress for your body shape, age, and lifestyle, so you can feel confident and comfortable in your own skin.

Body Shape

One of the most important things to consider when dressing is your body shape. Different body types will look better in different styles, cuts, and shapes of clothing. Here are some tips for dressing for your body shape:

1. Pear-shaped: If you have wider hips and a smaller waist, try wearing clothes that accentuate your waistline and draw attention to your upper body, such as wrap dresses, A-line skirts, and tops with interesting necklines.

2. Apple-shaped: If you carry more weight around your midsection, try wearing clothes that draw attention to your arms, legs, and bust, such as V-neck tops, A-line dresses, and high-waisted pants.

3. Hourglass-shaped: If you have a well-proportioned body with a defined waist, try wearing clothes that emphasize your curves, such as bodycon dresses, fitted tops, and high-waisted skirts.

4. Rectangle-shaped: If you have a straight-up-and-down body shape with little definition at the waist, try wearing clothes that create the illusion of curves, such as belted dresses, peplum tops, and wide-leg pants.

Age

Another factor to consider when dressing is your age. While there are no hard and fast rules about what you should wear at a certain age, there are some general guidelines that can help you look stylish and appropriate for your age. Here are some tips:

1. In your 20s: This is a time to experiment with different styles and trends, and have fun with fashion. Try bold prints, bright colors, and statement pieces.

2. In your 30s: This is a time to start investing in quality pieces that will last you for years to come. Look for classic, timeless styles that can be dressed up or down.

3. In your 40s: This is a time to focus on clothes that flatter your body shape and make you feel confident. Consider investing in good quality basics that you can mix and match.

4. In your 50s and beyond: This is a time to embrace your personal style and wear clothes that make you feel comfortable and confident. Look for classic pieces with a modern twist, and invest in good quality accessories.

Lifestyle

Your lifestyle is another important factor to consider when dressing. Your clothes should be functional and comfortable for your daily activities. Here are some tips for dressing for your lifestyle:

1. Office wear: If you work in a professional setting, your clothes should be polished and put-together. Look for tailored pieces, such as blazers, trousers, and pencil skirts.

2. Casual wear: If you have a more relaxed lifestyle, such as working from home or running errands, your clothes should be comfortable and easy to wear. Look for casual pieces, such as leggings, jeans, and T-shirts.

3. Athletic wear: If you enjoy working out or participating in sports, your clothes should be breathable and comfortable. Look for athletic wear, such as leggings, sports bras, and moisture-wicking tops.

In conclusion, dressing for your body shape, age, and lifestyle can help you feel confident and comfortable in your own skin. By following these tips, you can choose clothes that fl

3.3.3 - Cultivating a timeless, age-appropriate wardrobe

As we age, our personal style and wardrobe choices often change. The clothing that once looked great on us may no longer flatter our changing bodies, and our tastes and preferences may evolve over time. It's important to cultivate a wardrobe that not only makes us feel good but also reflects our age and lifestyle.

In this chapter, we'll explore some tips for creating a timeless, age-appropriate wardrobe that is both stylish and functional.

1. Invest in quality basics: Building a wardrobe of quality basics such as a well-fitting pair of jeans, a classic white shirt, and a

versatile blazer can serve as the foundation for any age-appropriate wardrobe. These timeless pieces can be dressed up or down and never go out of style.

2. Consider fit: It's important to dress for the body you have now and not the one you used to have or hope to have in the future. Clothing that is too tight or too loose can be unflattering and can add years to your appearance. Always opt for clothing that fits well and flatters your current body shape.

3. Choose classic prints and colors: Prints and colors that are classic and timeless are always in style. Opt for neutral colors like black, white, navy, and beige, and classic prints like stripes and polka dots.

4. Accessorize wisely: Accessories can take any outfit to the next level, but it's important not to overdo it. Choose statement pieces that are age-appropriate and pair them with more classic accessories.

5. Don't be afraid to try something new: While it's important to stick with what works for you, don't be afraid to try something new. Experiment with different styles, colors, and prints until you find what works for you.

6. Consider your lifestyle: Your wardrobe should reflect your lifestyle. If you are retired or work from home, you may not need as many formal pieces as someone who works in a corporate office. Consider your daily activities and build your wardrobe accordingly.

7. Embrace comfort: Comfortable clothing doesn't have to mean sloppy or unflattering. Opt for comfortable, yet stylish pieces that you feel good in and can move around comfortably in.

In conclusion, cultivating a timeless, age-appropriate wardrobe is all about investing in quality basics, choosing classic prints and colors, accessorizing wisely, trying something new, considering your lifestyle, and embracing comfort. By following these tips, you can create a wardrobe that makes you feel confident, stylish, and age-appropriate.

3.3.4 - The role of accessories and personal grooming in expressing individuality

The way we dress and present ourselves to the world can be a powerful tool for self-expression and communication. Accessories and personal grooming are key elements in creating a unique style that reflects our individuality and personality. In this chapter, we will explore the importance of accessories and personal grooming in creating a personal style that is both functional and expressive.

Accessories are a crucial part of any outfit. They can add a pop of color or texture, create interest and depth, and bring an outfit together. Accessories can be anything from jewelry, scarves, hats, belts, and bags, to shoes and even eyewear. Each accessory has its own unique purpose and can help create a cohesive look.

When choosing accessories, it's important to consider the overall style and color palette of your outfit. Neutral accessories can be versatile and work well with a variety of outfits, while bold accessories can add a touch of personality and create a statement look. It's important to strike a balance between functionality and style, ensuring that accessories not only look good but also serve a practical purpose.

Jewelry is one of the most popular accessories, and it can range from dainty and delicate to bold and statement-making. Necklaces, bracelets, earrings, and rings can all be used to add interest to an outfit. When choosing jewelry, consider the neckline of your outfit, the shape of your face, and your personal style. Some people prefer minimalistic jewelry, while others prefer bolder and more colorful pieces. Don't be afraid to experiment and find what works best for you.

Scarves and hats are also great accessories that can be used to add interest to an outfit. Scarves come in a variety of colors, patterns, and fabrics, and can be worn in different ways. They can be used to add warmth in cooler months or as a statement accessory in the summer. Hats are also versatile and can be used to complete an outfit, add a touch of personality, or protect from the sun.

Belts and bags are functional accessories that can also add style to an outfit. A belt can be used to cinch a dress or add structure to an oversized top, while a bag can be used to carry essentials and complete an outfit. When choosing a bag, consider its size, shape, and color. A bag should be functional and complement your outfit, rather than overpower it.

Personal grooming is another important aspect of personal style. It can refer to everything from hair and makeup to skincare and nail care. Personal grooming is a way to take care of ourselves and present our best selves to the world. A good grooming routine can also be a form of self-care and help boost confidence.

Hair is a key aspect of personal grooming, and there are many ways to style and care for it. Choosing a hairstyle that suits your face shape, hair type, and personal style can help create a cohesive look. Regular haircuts and treatments can also help maintain healthy hair.

Makeup is another tool for self-expression and can range from natural and minimalistic to bold and colorful. Makeup can be used to enhance features, create a flawless complexion, and add color and dimension. When choosing makeup, consider your skin type, personal style, and the occasion.

Skincare is an essential aspect of personal grooming, and a good skincare routine can help maintain healthy and youthful-looking skin. This can include cleansing, exfoliating, moisturizing, and using sunscreen. Skincare products should be chosen based on skin type and concerns.

Nail care is another important aspect of personal grooming. Regular manicures and pedicures can help keep nails healthy and strong. Nail polish can also be used to add color and personality to an outfit.

3.4: Rest, Relaxation, and Self-Care Rituals

3.4.1 - The importance of self-care in promoting health and longevity

Self-care is the practice of taking care of one's own physical, mental, and emotional health. It involves making intentional choices to promote well-being and prevent illness or disease. Self-care is not a one-time event but rather a lifelong process. The benefits of self-care are numerous, and it can lead to a better quality of life and increased longevity.

Importance of Self-Care:

Self-care is essential for maintaining good health and well-being. It allows individuals to take control of their health and make conscious decisions about their lifestyles. By practicing self-care, individuals can reduce their risk of developing chronic diseases, such as diabetes, heart disease, and cancer.

Self-care also promotes mental and emotional health. It can help individuals manage stress and prevent burnout. It allows individuals to prioritize their needs and take time for themselves, which can lead to improved mood and a better overall outlook on life.

Additionally, self-care can improve relationships with others. When individuals take care of themselves, they are better equipped to care for others. Self-care can also increase self-esteem and confidence, which can lead to better communication and stronger relationships.

Practicing Self-Care:

There are many ways to practice self-care, and individuals should choose activities that work for them. Some common self-care practices include:

1. Physical exercise: Regular physical activity is essential for maintaining good health. Exercise can improve cardiovascular health, strengthen muscles and bones, and improve mental health.

2. Eating a healthy diet: A nutritious diet is essential for maintaining good health. Eating a variety of fruits, vegetables, whole grains, lean proteins, and healthy fats can provide the body with essential nutrients.

3. Getting enough sleep: Sleep is essential for physical and mental health. Getting adequate sleep can improve mood, increase energy levels, and reduce the risk of developing chronic diseases.

4. Practicing mindfulness: Mindfulness is the practice of being present in the moment and paying attention to one's thoughts and feelings. Mindfulness can reduce stress, improve mental health, and increase overall well-being.

5. Engaging in hobbies and activities: Engaging in hobbies and activities that bring joy and fulfillment can improve mental and emotional health. Hobbies can reduce stress, increase creativity, and provide a sense of accomplishment.

Conclusion:

Self-care is an essential practice for promoting health and well-being. It involves making intentional choices to prioritize one's physical, mental, and emotional health. By practicing self-care, individuals can improve their quality of life, prevent chronic diseases, and promote longevity. There are many ways to practice self-care, and individuals should choose activities that work for them.

3.4.2 - Techniques for managing stress and finding balance

In today's fast-paced world, stress is a common issue that affects many people. It can lead to a wide range of health problems, both physical and mental. That's why it's important to manage stress and find balance in life. In this chapter, we'll explore some techniques that can help you manage stress and achieve balance.

One effective technique for managing stress is mindfulness meditation. This involves focusing your attention on the present moment and accepting your thoughts and feelings without judgment. Studies have shown that mindfulness meditation can reduce symptoms of anxiety and depression, lower cortisol levels, and improve overall well-being.

Another technique for managing stress is physical activity. Exercise can help reduce stress by releasing endorphins, which are natural mood boosters. It can also improve sleep quality, reduce inflammation, and lower blood pressure.

It's also important to make time for relaxation and self-care. This can involve activities such as taking a hot bath, getting a massage, or spending time in nature. These activities can help you reduce stress and promote feelings of calmness and relaxation.

Finally, finding balance in life means making time for the things that matter most to you. This could be spending time with loved ones, pursuing a hobby, or volunteering in your community. By finding balance and making time for the things that bring you joy, you can reduce stress and improve your overall quality of life.

In summary, managing stress and finding balance in life is essential for promoting health and longevity. Mindfulness meditation, physical activity, relaxation and self-care, and making time for the things that matter most to you are all effective techniques for achieving this goal.

3.4.3 - The benefits of regular self-care rituals and practices

Self-care is a term that has been gaining popularity in recent years, and for good reason. It refers to the practice of taking care of one's own physical, mental, and emotional health. Engaging in self-care activities can help individuals maintain balance and prevent burnout, as well as promote overall health and well-being.

Self-care is not a one-size-fits-all approach. It's important to find activities that work for you and incorporate them into your routine. Below are some examples of self-care practices that can provide a wide range of benefits.

1. Mindfulness and Meditation: Mindfulness and meditation are practices that involve being present in the moment and

focusing on breathing, thoughts, and sensations. These practices have been shown to reduce stress, improve sleep, and increase feelings of calm and well-being.

2. Exercise: Regular exercise has numerous physical and mental health benefits, including reducing the risk of chronic diseases, improving mood, and reducing stress and anxiety.

3. Journaling: Writing down thoughts and feelings can be a helpful tool for processing emotions and reducing stress. It can also be a way to track progress and reflect on personal growth.

4. Social Support: Spending time with friends and loved ones can help reduce feelings of loneliness and improve mood. Engaging in hobbies or activities with others can provide a sense of community and support.

5. Creative Expression: Engaging in creative activities, such as painting, drawing, or writing, can provide an outlet for emotions and reduce stress. It can also be a way to explore personal interests and passions.

6. Sleep: Getting enough quality sleep is crucial for overall health and well-being. Poor sleep has been linked to a variety of health issues, including weight gain, weakened immune system, and decreased cognitive function.

Incorporating self-care practices into your routine can have a profound impact on your overall health and well-being. It's important to remember that self-care is not selfish or indulgent, but rather an essential part of maintaining a healthy and balanced life.

3.4.4 - Creating a personalized self-care plan to nurture body, mind, and spirit

Self-care refers to the act of taking care of oneself physically, emotionally, and mentally. It is essential for maintaining good health, reducing stress, and promoting overall well-being. In this chapter, we will explore the importance of self-care and how it can be used to promote health and longevity. We will also discuss different techniques for managing stress and finding balance, as well as the benefits of regular self-care rituals and practices. Finally, we will provide guidance on creating a personalized self-care plan to nurture the body, mind, and spirit.

The Importance of Self-Care:

Self-care is an essential component of a healthy lifestyle. It involves taking time to care for yourself and your needs, both physically and mentally. Practicing self-care can reduce stress, increase energy levels, and promote better sleep. It also helps to prevent burnout and improves overall well-being.

Stress Management and Finding Balance:

Stress is a common problem in today's fast-paced society. It can have negative effects on both physical and mental health. Therefore, it is important to have techniques for managing stress and finding balance in life. This can include activities like exercise, meditation, spending time in nature, and engaging in hobbies or activities that bring joy and fulfillment.

The Benefits of Regular Self-Care Rituals and Practices:

Regular self-care rituals and practices can provide many benefits for overall well-being. They can help to reduce stress, improve sleep, and increase feelings of self-worth and confidence. Some examples of self-care rituals include taking a relaxing bath, practicing yoga or meditation, or engaging in a creative activity.

Creating a Personalized Self-Care Plan:

Creating a personalized self-care plan involves identifying your individual needs and developing a plan that addresses them. This can include setting aside time for exercise, planning healthy meals, scheduling time for hobbies or self-care activities, and practicing stress-management techniques. It is important to prioritize self-care as an essential component of a healthy lifestyle.

Conclusion:

Self-care is an essential component of a healthy lifestyle. It involves taking time to care for oneself physically, emotionally, and mentally. Practicing self-care can reduce stress, increase energy levels, and promote overall well-being. By implementing self-care rituals and practices, and developing a personalized self-care plan, individuals can take control of their health and well-being, and improve their quality of life.

Chapter 4: Embracing the Journey: A Roadmap for Longevity and Fulfillment

4.1: Setting Goals and Embracing Change

4.1.1 - The importance of goal setting and personal growth for lifelong fulfillment

Chapter 4.1.1 - The Importance of Goal Setting and Personal Growth for Lifelong Fulfillment

The human journey is one of constant growth and development, and the pursuit of fulfillment is an integral part of this process. While the definition of fulfillment varies from person to person, it is safe to say that it involves the pursuit of happiness, joy, and contentment in all aspects of life. Achieving fulfillment requires intentional effort, self-awareness, and a willingness to challenge oneself. In this chapter, we will explore the importance of goal setting and personal growth in attaining lifelong fulfillment.

Goal Setting

Goals provide direction and purpose in life. They help us focus on what is truly important and enable us to take concrete steps towards achieving our desired outcomes. Goals can be short-term or long-term, and they can pertain to any area of life, including career, relationships, health, personal growth, and financial stability.

The process of setting goals involves identifying what we want to achieve and then developing a plan to make it happen. Goals should be specific, measurable, achievable, relevant, and time-bound. This is often referred to as the SMART goal-setting framework. When we set SMART goals, we are more likely to achieve them because they are realistic, tangible, and within our control.

Personal Growth

Personal growth is the process of self-improvement and self-discovery. It involves developing new skills, expanding one's knowledge, and increasing self-awareness. Personal growth is an ongoing journey that requires a commitment to learning, reflection, and growth.

One of the most effective ways to pursue personal growth is through intentional learning. This can take many forms, such as reading books, attending workshops or seminars, taking online courses, or seeking mentorship from someone with more experience. Engaging in intentional learning helps us expand our knowledge, develop new skills, and gain a deeper understanding of ourselves and the world around us.

Another important aspect of personal growth is self-reflection. Self-reflection involves examining our thoughts, feelings, and behaviors to gain insight into our strengths, weaknesses, and areas for improvement. It helps us identify patterns in our behavior and thought processes, and it enables us to make positive changes in our lives.

Benefits of Goal Setting and Personal Growth

The pursuit of goal setting and personal growth has many benefits. It can lead to increased self-awareness, improved confidence and self-esteem, and greater resilience in the face of challenges. It can also help us develop stronger relationships, achieve greater success in our careers, and experience a greater sense of purpose and fulfillment in life.

Goal setting and personal growth also provide a sense of direction and purpose. When we have a clear sense of what we want to achieve and how we want to grow, we are more likely to stay focused and motivated. This can help us overcome obstacles and setbacks along the way.

Conclusion

Goal setting and personal growth are essential components of a fulfilling life. By setting specific, measurable, achievable, relevant, and time-bound goals, we can pursue our desired outcomes with intention and purpose. Engaging in intentional learning and self-reflection can help us develop new skills, expand our knowledge, and gain a deeper understanding of ourselves and the world around us. The pursuit of goal setting and personal growth can lead to increased self-awareness, improved confidence and self-esteem, and greater resilience in the face of challenges, ultimately leading to a more fulfilling life.

4.1.2 - Overcoming obstacles and adapting to life's inevitable changes

Life is full of challenges and obstacles, and it is important to learn how to overcome them to achieve personal growth and lifelong fulfillment. Change is also an inevitable part of life, and learning to adapt to it can help us navigate through life's ups and downs with greater ease.

Obstacles and challenges can take many forms, such as health issues, financial difficulties, relationship problems, career setbacks, and more. However, it is important to remember that these challenges can also present opportunities for personal growth and learning. By facing and overcoming obstacles, we can develop resilience, confidence, and a sense of accomplishment that can help us in all areas of life.

To overcome obstacles, it is important to have a positive mindset and a willingness to take action. Here are some tips for overcoming obstacles:

1. Identify the problem: The first step in overcoming an obstacle is to identify the problem and understand what is causing it. This can help you to develop a plan of action to address the issue.

2. Set realistic goals: Once you have identified the problem, set realistic goals that will help you to overcome it. These goals should be specific, measurable, and achievable.

3. Take action: Taking action is essential to overcoming obstacles. This may involve seeking advice from others,

learning new skills, or making changes to your lifestyle or habits.

4. Stay focused: Staying focused on your goals can help you to maintain a positive mindset and stay motivated to overcome obstacles. It can also help to break down your goals into smaller, more manageable steps.

5. Celebrate your successes: Celebrating your successes, no matter how small, can help you to stay motivated and focused on achieving your goals.

Adapting to life's changes is also an important skill to develop. Change can come in many forms, such as moving to a new city, changing jobs, or experiencing a loss or a major life transition. Adapting to change requires flexibility, resilience, and a willingness to embrace new experiences and challenges.

Here are some tips for adapting to life's changes:

1. Stay positive: Maintaining a positive attitude can help you to stay resilient and open to new experiences.

2. Embrace the change: Embracing change can help you to see new opportunities and possibilities that you may not have considered before.

3. Be flexible: Being flexible and adaptable can help you to navigate unexpected changes and challenges with greater ease.

4. Seek support: Seeking support from family, friends, or professionals can help you to navigate through difficult transitions and changes.

5. Take care of yourself: Taking care of yourself physically, mentally, and emotionally can help you to build resilience and adapt to life's changes with greater ease.

In conclusion, overcoming obstacles and adapting to life's changes are important skills to develop for personal growth and lifelong fulfillment. By approaching challenges with a positive mindset and a willingness to take action, and by staying flexible and open to new experiences, we can navigate through life's ups and downs with greater ease and achieve our goals.

4.1.3 - The power of perseverance and resilience in the face of adversity

Life is full of challenges and setbacks that can cause us to feel overwhelmed and defeated. Whether it's a personal loss, a professional setback, or a health issue, adversity can be difficult to face. However, developing the ability to persevere and bounce back from adversity is an essential skill for living a fulfilling and successful life. In this chapter, we will explore the power of perseverance and resilience in the face of adversity and provide strategies for cultivating these traits.

Perseverance is the ability to persist in the face of obstacles and setbacks. It's the determination to keep going, even when things get tough. Resilience, on the other hand, is the ability to recover quickly from adversity and to adapt to change.

Together, these traits enable us to overcome challenges and achieve our goals, even when the odds are against us.

There are many benefits to developing perseverance and resilience. For one, these traits help us to stay focused on our goals, even in the face of distractions and setbacks. They also help us to bounce back from failure and disappointment, enabling us to learn from our mistakes and move forward. In addition, perseverance and resilience can help us to maintain a positive outlook and a sense of hope, even in difficult times.

So how can we cultivate these traits? Here are some strategies to consider:

1. Develop a growth mindset: A growth mindset is the belief that we can improve our abilities through hard work and persistence. When we adopt a growth mindset, we are more likely to see obstacles as opportunities for growth and to view failure as a natural part of the learning process.

2. Focus on what you can control: In any situation, there are things we can control and things we can't. By focusing on what we can control, such as our own thoughts and actions, we can maintain a sense of agency and reduce feelings of helplessness.

3. Practice self-care: Taking care of ourselves is essential for maintaining resilience. This includes getting enough sleep, eating a healthy diet, and engaging in regular exercise. It also means taking time for activities that bring us joy and relaxation, such as reading a book, listening to music, or spending time with loved ones.

4. Seek support: No one can face adversity alone. It's important to seek out support from friends, family, or a professional counselor. Talking about our problems can help us gain perspective and find solutions.

5. Learn from adversity: Adversity can be a powerful teacher. By reflecting on our experiences and what we have learned from them, we can develop a greater sense of wisdom and resilience.

In conclusion, developing the ability to persevere and bounce back from adversity is an essential skill for living a fulfilling and successful life. By cultivating a growth mindset, focusing on what we can control, practicing self-care, seeking support, and learning from adversity, we can develop the resilience needed to overcome life's challenges and achieve our goals.

4.1.4 - Achieving balance and success in all areas of life

When we think of success, we often focus on our professional achievements. But true success is about achieving balance and fulfillment in all areas of life. This includes our relationships, health, personal growth, and leisure activities.

The first step to achieving balance and success is to set goals in each area of life. This will give us direction and help us prioritize our time and resources. However, it's important to set realistic goals and to be flexible as we adapt to new circumstances.

In order to achieve balance, we must also learn to manage our time effectively. This means prioritizing tasks and learning to say "no" to activities that are not aligned with our goals. It also means taking breaks and practicing self-care to avoid burnout.

Another key to achieving balance and success is to cultivate positive relationships. This includes our relationships with family, friends, colleagues, and community. We must learn to communicate effectively, listen actively, and be supportive of one another.

In addition to positive relationships, we must also prioritize our health. This includes getting enough sleep, exercise, and proper nutrition. It also means practicing stress-reducing activities such as meditation and mindfulness.

Finally, we must make time for leisure activities that bring us joy and fulfillment. This could include hobbies, travel, or volunteering. Taking time for these activities can help us recharge and avoid burnout.

Achieving balance and success in all areas of life is not easy, but it is possible with dedication and effort. By setting realistic goals, managing our time effectively, cultivating positive relationships, prioritizing our health, and making time for leisure activities, we can achieve fulfillment and balance in our lives.

4.2: Lifelong Learning and Exploration

4.2.1 - The benefits of continuous learning for cognitive health and personal growth

Learning is a lifelong process, and it has many benefits beyond just acquiring knowledge. In fact, continuous learning is essential for cognitive health and personal growth. Whether it's learning a new language, a musical instrument, or a new skill, continuous learning can help keep the brain active and healthy, improve memory and concentration, and even help stave off cognitive decline in later life. Moreover, learning can also provide a sense of purpose and fulfillment, and can open up new opportunities for personal and professional growth.

The Importance of Continuous Learning for Cognitive Health:

Learning stimulates the brain and helps keep it active, which is crucial for maintaining cognitive health. As we age, our brain cells begin to die, and our brain's ability to form new connections and adapt to changing circumstances slows down. However, learning new things can help to counteract this decline and keep the brain healthy and functioning at its best. Studies have shown that regular learning and mental stimulation can reduce the risk of cognitive decline, dementia, and other age-related cognitive impairments.

Learning new things also helps to improve memory and concentration, as it challenges the brain to create and retain new information. Learning a new language, for example, can help improve cognitive function, as it requires the brain to process and retain new vocabulary, grammar, and syntax. Similarly, learning a musical instrument or a new skill can help improve hand-eye coordination, focus, and attention to detail.

The Benefits of Continuous Learning for Personal Growth:

Continuous learning also has many benefits for personal growth and development. Learning new things can provide a sense of purpose and fulfillment, as it allows us to pursue our interests and passions. It can also help us develop new skills and talents, and can open up new opportunities for personal and professional growth.

Learning can also help us to become more adaptable and resilient, as it teaches us how to approach new challenges and adapt to changing circumstances. It can help us develop problem-solving skills and creative thinking, as we learn to think outside the box and explore new ideas and perspectives.

Strategies for Continuous Learning:

There are many ways to incorporate continuous learning into our lives, no matter our age or interests. Here are some strategies for continuous learning:

1. Take an online course or enroll in a class in a subject you're interested in.

2. Join a book club or attend lectures and events on topics you're curious about.

3. Learn a new language or a musical instrument.

4. Volunteer for a new project or job that requires you to learn new skills.

5. Attend workshops and seminars to learn about new trends and developments in your field.

6. Read books and articles on a wide range of topics to expand your knowledge and perspectives.

7. Try new hobbies or activities that challenge you to learn new skills.

Conclusion:

Continuous learning is essential for cognitive health and personal growth. It helps keep the brain active and healthy, improves memory and concentration, and provides a sense of purpose and fulfillment. Whether it's learning a new language, a musical instrument, or a new skill, there are many ways to incorporate continuous learning into our lives. By making continuous learning a priority, we can unlock our full potential and lead fulfilling and meaningful lives.

4.2.2 - Strategies for lifelong learning and intellectual curiosity

In today's fast-paced world, it is more important than ever to stay engaged and curious about the world around us. One of the best ways to do this is through lifelong learning. Continuously acquiring new knowledge and skills can not only boost cognitive health but also lead to personal growth and fulfillment. In this chapter, we will explore the benefits of continuous learning and strategies for staying engaged and curious throughout life.

The Benefits of Continuous Learning:

Continuous learning can have a multitude of benefits, including:

1. Cognitive Health: Learning new things can stimulate the brain and improve cognitive function. Research has shown that lifelong learning can help to prevent cognitive decline and reduce the risk of developing diseases such as dementia.

2. Personal Growth: Learning new things can help us to expand our perspectives, challenge our assumptions, and grow as individuals. It can also lead to increased creativity and innovation.

3. Career Advancement: Continuous learning can help us to stay current in our fields and develop new skills that can lead to career advancement and opportunities.

4. Social Connection: Learning can also be a social activity, providing opportunities to connect with others who share our interests and passions.

Strategies for Lifelong Learning:

Here are some strategies for staying engaged and curious throughout life:

1. Pursue Your Interests: Learning is most enjoyable when it is something that we are interested in. Identify your passions and pursue them through reading, taking classes, attending workshops, or joining a community group.

2. Embrace Technology: Technology has made learning more accessible than ever. Take advantage of online courses, podcasts, and educational apps to learn on the go.

3. Learn From Others: Learning doesn't always have to be self-directed. Seek out mentors, attend conferences, and participate in group learning activities to learn from others and build connections.

4. Stay Open-Minded: To truly benefit from learning, it's important to approach new ideas and experiences with an open mind. Be willing to challenge your assumptions and consider new perspectives.

Conclusion:

Continuous learning is a valuable practice that can lead to improved cognitive health, personal growth, and career advancement. By pursuing our interests, embracing technology, learning from others, and staying open-minded, we can stay engaged and curious throughout our lives.

4.2.3 - Embracing creativity, innovation, and new experiences

Introduction

In today's fast-paced world, it is essential to stay ahead of the curve and continuously evolve. This requires an open mind, a willingness to learn and grow, and an ability to embrace creativity, innovation, and new experiences. In this chapter, we will explore the importance of these traits and how they can help you achieve personal growth and fulfillment.

The Importance of Creativity

Creativity is not just a trait reserved for artists and musicians. It is a crucial component of success in all areas of life, from business to personal relationships. Creativity allows us to think outside the box, come up with new solutions to old problems, and find innovative ways to tackle challenges.

One of the best ways to cultivate creativity is to allow yourself to be curious and explore new ideas. Try new hobbies, read books on different subjects, and expose yourself to diverse perspectives. Additionally, taking time to reflect and letting your mind wander can help you come up with fresh and innovative ideas.

The Benefits of Innovation

Innovation is the act of taking creative ideas and turning them into tangible solutions. It is the driving force behind progress and growth, both on a personal and societal level. Innovation allows us to find new ways of doing things, develop better products and services, and improve our overall quality of life.

To be innovative, it is important to stay informed about new developments in your field or industry, seek out feedback and input from others, and be willing to take calculated risks. It is also crucial to maintain a positive attitude and a growth mindset, always looking for ways to improve and enhance your work.

The Value of New Experiences

New experiences can be intimidating, but they are also incredibly valuable for personal growth and development.

Whether it is traveling to a new place, trying a new hobby, or meeting new people, stepping out of your comfort zone can broaden your horizons and give you a fresh perspective on life.

To make the most of new experiences, it is important to approach them with an open mind and a willingness to learn. Take the time to reflect on what you have learned and how it has impacted your perspective. This will help you grow and evolve as a person and be better equipped to handle new challenges in the future.

Conclusion

In conclusion, embracing creativity, innovation, and new experiences is essential for personal growth and fulfillment. By cultivating these traits, you can stay ahead of the curve, find new solutions to old problems, and expand your horizons in ways you never thought possible. So, don't be afraid to think outside the box, take calculated risks, and explore new opportunities. Your future self will thank you.

4.2.4 - The role of travel and cultural exploration in fostering a rich, meaningful life

In today's fast-paced world, it's easy to get caught up in the daily grind and forget about the importance of personal growth and exploration. However, continuous learning and seeking out new experiences can have numerous benefits, from improving cognitive health to increasing overall happiness and fulfillment in life. In this chapter, we will explore the many ways in which lifelong learning, creativity, and cultural exploration can help us lead richer, more meaningful lives.

Section 1: The Benefits of Continuous Learning

Continuous learning refers to the practice of consistently seeking out new knowledge and skills throughout our lives. This can take many forms, such as taking classes, attending seminars, or simply reading books and articles on new topics. But why is continuous learning so important? Here are some of the benefits:

1. Improved Cognitive Health: Studies have shown that engaging in mentally stimulating activities, such as reading or learning a new skill, can help improve cognitive function and reduce the risk of cognitive decline and dementia in older age.

2. Increased Creativity: Learning new things can help stimulate creativity by exposing us to new ideas and perspectives. This can translate into increased innovation and problem-solving abilities in other areas of our lives.

3. Increased Confidence: When we take the initiative to learn something new, we gain a sense of accomplishment and confidence in our abilities, which can translate into other areas of our lives.

4. Improved Career Prospects: Continuous learning can help us stay up-to-date with the latest developments in our field and improve our job performance, leading to potential career advancements and opportunities.

Section 2: Strategies for Lifelong Learning and Intellectual Curiosity

While the benefits of continuous learning are clear, it can be difficult to know where to start. Here are some strategies for fostering a lifelong love of learning:

1. Set Goals: Identify areas in which you would like to improve or learn more about, and set specific goals for yourself. This can help keep you motivated and focused on your learning journey.

2. Stay Curious: Cultivate a sense of curiosity about the world around you. Ask questions, seek out new experiences, and never stop learning.

3. Embrace Technology: In today's digital age, there are countless resources available online for learning new skills and subjects. Take advantage of these resources, such as online courses and tutorials.

4. Stay Accountable: Share your learning goals with others and hold yourself accountable for your progress. Join a learning group or find an accountability partner to help keep you motivated.

Section 3: Embracing Creativity, Innovation, and New Experiences

Creativity and innovation are essential for personal growth and development. Here are some ways to embrace these qualities in your life:

1. Pursue Hobbies: Engage in activities that allow you to express your creativity, such as painting, writing, or playing

music. These activities can help you relax and de-stress while also stimulating your mind.

2. Take Risks: Be willing to try new things and take risks, even if they are outside your comfort zone. This can help you develop new skills and expand your perspective.

3. Collaborate with Others: Working with others can spark new ideas and inspire creativity. Consider joining a group or team focused on a shared interest or project.

Section 4: The Role of Travel and Cultural Exploration

Travel and cultural exploration can be transformative experiences that broaden our horizons and expose us to new perspectives and ways of life. Here are some of the benefits:

1. Increased Empathy: Experiencing different cultures can help us develop empathy and understanding for people from different backgrounds and walks of life.

2. Personal Growth: Travel and cultural exploration can challenge us to step outside our comfort zones, leading to personal growth and development.

3. New Perspectives: Exposure to new cultures and ways of life can help us

4.3: Leaving a Legacy: Contributions to Future Generations

4.3.1 - The importance of leaving a positive impact on the world

As humans, we are not meant to live in isolation. Our actions and choices have an impact on the people and the world around us. In this chapter, we will explore the importance of leaving a positive impact on the world and the various ways in which we can do so.

Leaving a positive impact on the world means making a difference in the lives of others, contributing to the greater good, and leaving the world a better place than we found it. It is about creating a legacy that will be remembered long after we are gone.

One way to leave a positive impact on the world is through acts of kindness and generosity. Simple acts like volunteering at a local shelter, donating to a charitable organization, or helping a neighbor in need can make a significant difference in someone's life. These small acts of kindness have a ripple effect and can inspire others to do the same.

Another way to leave a positive impact on the world is through environmental conservation. By reducing our carbon footprint, conserving water, and protecting natural resources, we can contribute to a healthier and more sustainable planet for future generations. This can be done through small changes in our daily lives, such as using reusable bags and water bottles, conserving energy, and reducing waste.

Education and advocacy are also important ways to leave a positive impact on the world. By educating ourselves and others about important issues, we can raise awareness and promote positive change. Advocacy involves using our voices to support causes and policies that promote equality, justice, and human rights. Through education and advocacy, we can create a more informed and compassionate society.

Finally, living a life of purpose and fulfillment can leave a positive impact on the world. By pursuing our passions and doing what we love, we can inspire others to do the same and create a ripple effect of positivity and passion. This can involve pursuing a career in a field we are passionate about, volunteering in our community, or simply living a life that aligns with our values and beliefs.

In conclusion, leaving a positive impact on the world is essential to living a meaningful and fulfilling life. Whether through acts of kindness, environmental conservation, education and advocacy, or living a life of purpose and fulfillment, we can all make a difference in the world and create a legacy that will be remembered for generations to come.

4.3.2 - Identifying your unique strengths and passions for creating a meaningful legacy

Living a meaningful life is something that many people aspire to. One of the ways to achieve this is by leaving a positive impact on the world. This impact could be through making a difference in the lives of those around us or in the wider community. To do this, it is important to identify our unique strengths and passions so that we can use them to create a lasting legacy.

Identifying your strengths:

Strengths are the things we are naturally good at or have a talent for. They are the things that come easily to us and that we enjoy doing. Identifying your strengths is an important step in creating a meaningful legacy as it allows you to use them to make a positive impact. Here are some tips for identifying your strengths:

1. Look at what comes naturally to you: Think about the things that come easily to you, and that you enjoy doing. These could be skills such as problem-solving, communication, or creativity.

2. Ask for feedback: Sometimes we are not aware of our strengths, but others around us may have noticed them. Ask for feedback from friends, family, or colleagues to help identify your strengths.

3. Reflect on your past successes: Think about times when you have achieved success in your life. What strengths did you use to achieve that success?

4. Take a strengths assessment: There are many online assessments that can help you identify your strengths. These can provide valuable insights into your unique abilities and talents.

Identifying your passions:

Passions are the things we are deeply interested in and care about. They are the things that give us a sense of purpose and meaning. Identifying your passions is important as it allows you to focus your efforts on something that is meaningful to you. Here are some tips for identifying your passions:

1. Think about what excites you: Consider the things that you enjoy doing in your free time. What hobbies or activities do you find most enjoyable?

2. Consider your values: Our passions often align with our values. Think about the things that are most important to you, such as family, community, or social justice.

3. Reflect on your life experiences: Our life experiences can often shape our passions. Think about the experiences that have had the most impact on you and what passions may have arisen from those experiences.

4. Explore new things: Sometimes we may not know what our passions are until we try new things. Be open to new experiences and try new hobbies or activities to see what resonates with you.

Creating a meaningful legacy:

Once you have identified your unique strengths and passions, it is important to use them to create a lasting impact on the world. Here are some tips for creating a meaningful legacy:

1. Set goals: Identify specific goals that align with your strengths and passions. These could be anything from volunteering at a local charity to starting your own business.

2. Find a mentor: Seek out someone who has already made a positive impact in the area you are interested in. They can provide guidance and support as you work towards your goals.

3. Collaborate with others: Many meaningful legacies are created through collaboration. Partner with others who share your passions and strengths to achieve a greater impact.

4. Stay focused: Creating a meaningful legacy takes time and effort. Stay focused on your goals and stay committed to making a positive impact.

In conclusion, identifying your unique strengths and passions is an important step in creating a meaningful legacy. By using these to make a positive impact on the world, you can leave a lasting legacy that will inspire others to do the same.

4.3.3 - Mentoring and supporting the next generation: Sharing wisdom and experiences

As we age, we have the unique opportunity to share our wisdom and experiences with the next generation. Mentoring is a powerful way to pass on knowledge, skills, and values to younger people and contribute to their personal and professional growth. It is a way to make a meaningful impact on the world and leave a positive legacy.

Mentoring can take many forms, from informal conversations and guidance to more structured relationships, such as formal mentorship programs. Regardless of the form it takes, mentoring is a powerful way to give back and help others reach their potential.

Identifying Mentoring Opportunities

There are many ways to identify opportunities to mentor others. Consider volunteering with a local organization that supports young people or joining a mentorship program through your workplace or professional organization. You can also reach out to younger colleagues or acquaintances and offer to share your experience and insights with them.

Mentoring can also be a way to support individuals who have faced challenges or barriers in their lives. For example, you might consider mentoring someone who is transitioning out of foster care or who has been involved in the criminal justice system. By providing guidance and support, you can help them overcome obstacles and achieve their goals.

Sharing Your Experience and Insights

One of the most important aspects of mentoring is sharing your experience and insights with others. This can involve discussing challenges you faced in your career or personal life, sharing lessons you learned along the way, and offering advice on how to navigate difficult situations.

It is also important to listen actively to the mentee and help them identify their strengths, weaknesses, and goals.

Mentoring is a two-way street, and you can learn as much from your mentee as they can learn from you.

Building a Strong Mentoring Relationship

Building a strong mentoring relationship takes time and effort. It requires building trust, setting clear expectations, and establishing regular communication. It is important to be reliable and responsive, and to provide feedback and support as needed.

In addition to providing guidance and support, mentoring can also be a way to expand your own network and learn from others. Mentoring relationships can lead to new opportunities, collaborations, and friendships that can enrich your life and contribute to your own personal and professional growth.

Conclusion

Mentoring is a powerful way to give back and make a positive impact on the world. By sharing your wisdom, experience, and insights with the next generation, you can help them achieve their goals and contribute to their personal and professional growth. Mentoring can be a fulfilling and rewarding experience, and can leave a lasting legacy that extends far beyond your own lifetime.

4.3.4 - Philanthropy, volunteerism, and community involvement: Giving back to society

In today's world, giving back to society has become an important aspect of many people's lives. It is a way of expressing gratitude for the blessings received, as well as contributing towards making the world a better place. Philanthropy, volunteerism, and community involvement are all avenues for individuals to give back and make a difference in the lives of others. This chapter will explore the benefits of these activities and provide tips on how to get involved.

Benefits of Philanthropy, Volunteerism, and Community Involvement

1. Sense of Purpose and Fulfillment: When you give back to society, it provides a sense of purpose and fulfillment that cannot be found elsewhere. Helping others and making a difference in the lives of those in need can bring immense joy and satisfaction.

2. Personal Growth: Giving back allows individuals to learn new skills and experiences that can contribute to personal growth. Volunteering, for example, provides an opportunity to develop new talents, enhance communication skills, and improve teamwork.

3. Networking and Collaboration: Philanthropy, volunteerism, and community involvement are great ways to meet new people and build networks. Collaborating with others towards a common goal can lead to meaningful connections that can have a positive impact on both personal and professional lives.

4. Improved Mental and Physical Health: Engaging in philanthropy, volunteerism, and community involvement has been linked to improved mental and physical health. It can

reduce stress, boost self-esteem, and increase feelings of happiness and well-being.

Tips for Getting Involved

1. Identify Your Interests: The first step towards getting involved is to identify your interests. What causes or issues are you passionate about? This will help you choose organizations or initiatives that align with your values and beliefs.

2. Start Small: If you are new to giving back, start small by participating in a local charity event or fundraiser. This will allow you to dip your toes in the water and get a sense of what it's like to give back to society.

3. Do Your Research: Before getting involved with an organization, do your research. Learn about their mission, values, and programs to ensure that they align with your interests and goals.

4. Consider Your Skills and Resources: Think about the skills and resources you can offer an organization. Are you good at fundraising, event planning, or marketing? Can you offer your time or financial support? By leveraging your strengths, you can make a meaningful contribution.

5. Connect with Others: Joining a group or team can make giving back more fun and social. Consider volunteering with friends, family, or colleagues to make it a team effort.

Conclusion

Philanthropy, volunteerism, and community involvement are all important ways to give back and make a difference in the lives of others. Engaging in these activities can provide a sense of purpose, personal growth, and improved mental and physical health. By identifying your interests, starting small, doing your research, leveraging your skills and resources, and connecting with others, you can make a meaningful contribution and leave a positive impact on society.

4.4: Spirituality, Purpose, and Inner Peace

4.4.1 - The role of spirituality and faith in finding purpose and inner peace

Spirituality and faith have been an essential part of human culture for thousands of years. These concepts have been used to explain the unexplainable, provide hope in times of despair, and offer guidance in living a fulfilling life. While spirituality and faith are often associated with religion, they can also exist independently of any religious practice. In this chapter, we will explore the role of spirituality and faith in finding purpose and inner peace.

The Search for Purpose

The search for purpose is a fundamental aspect of the human experience. We all want to know that our lives have meaning and that we are contributing to something greater than ourselves. Many people turn to spirituality and faith as a way to find their purpose in life. This can involve exploring religious teachings, practicing meditation or mindfulness, or simply spending time in nature.

Spirituality and faith can offer a sense of connection to something greater than ourselves. This connection can provide a sense of purpose and direction in life. By focusing on our spiritual beliefs, we can gain clarity on our values, goals, and aspirations. This can help us prioritize what is truly important and make decisions that align with our purpose.

Finding Inner Peace

In today's fast-paced and often stressful world, finding inner peace can be a challenge. Many people turn to spirituality and faith as a way to find peace and tranquility in their lives. Through prayer, meditation, or simply spending time in quiet reflection, individuals can tap into a sense of calm and inner stillness.

Spirituality and faith can also offer a sense of hope and comfort during difficult times. Belief in a higher power or a greater purpose can provide a sense of perspective and help individuals navigate challenges with greater resilience.

Living a Meaningful Life

Ultimately, the goal of spirituality and faith is to live a meaningful and fulfilling life. By connecting with something greater than ourselves, we can find purpose, inner peace, and a sense of community. We can also cultivate compassion, gratitude, and forgiveness, which can improve our relationships and overall well-being.

Conclusion

Spirituality and faith can offer a valuable framework for finding purpose and inner peace in life. Whether through religious practice or independent spiritual exploration, individuals can tap into a sense of connection and find meaning in their lives. By cultivating a deeper understanding of our spiritual beliefs, we can live a more fulfilling and purpose-driven life.

4.4.2 - Cultivating a strong sense of purpose throughout life

A sense of purpose is a vital component of a fulfilling and meaningful life. It provides direction, motivation, and a sense of accomplishment. As we go through life, our sense of purpose may change or evolve, but having a clear understanding of what we want to achieve and why is essential to our overall well-being.

Defining Purpose

Purpose can be defined as a reason for existing or a sense of direction in life. It can manifest in different ways, such as a specific goal, a sense of mission, or a desire to make a positive impact on the world. A strong sense of purpose is linked to better mental and physical health, increased happiness and life satisfaction, and greater resilience in the face of challenges.

Finding Your Purpose

Finding your purpose can be a lifelong journey, and it may take time and reflection to discover what truly drives you. Some helpful questions to ask yourself include:

- What are my values and beliefs?

- What am I passionate about?

- What are my strengths and talents?

- What impact do I want to have on the world?

- What brings me joy and fulfillment?

It can also be helpful to seek guidance from trusted friends or family members, a mentor or coach, or a therapist or counselor. They can provide support and offer valuable insights as you explore your purpose.

Cultivating Purpose

Once you have identified your purpose, it's important to cultivate it and integrate it into your daily life. Some ways to do this include:

- Setting goals that align with your purpose

- Seeking out opportunities that allow you to pursue your purpose

- Finding ways to use your strengths and talents in service of your purpose

- Surrounding yourself with people who support and encourage your purpose

- Maintaining a sense of gratitude for the opportunities to live out your purpose

Challenges to Purpose

There may be times when our sense of purpose is challenged, such as during periods of transition, setbacks, or loss. It's important to remember that setbacks and challenges are a natural part of the journey and can even provide opportunities for growth and development. Staying connected to our values and beliefs, seeking support from others, and maintaining a growth mindset can help us navigate these challenges and stay focused on our purpose.

Conclusion

Cultivating a strong sense of purpose throughout life can provide a sense of direction, motivation, and fulfillment. By exploring our values, passions, strengths, and goals, we can identify our purpose and integrate it into our daily lives. Despite challenges and setbacks, maintaining a sense of purpose can help us stay focused on what truly matters and lead a fulfilling life.

4.4.3 - Practices for fostering inner peace and emotional well-being

In today's fast-paced and demanding world, it is easy to get caught up in stress, anxiety, and negativity. To achieve a fulfilling and meaningful life, it is essential to take care of our emotional well-being and cultivate inner peace. This chapter will explore some practices and strategies for fostering inner peace and emotional well-being.

1. Mindfulness Meditation

Mindfulness meditation is a powerful tool for calming the mind and promoting emotional well-being. It involves focusing your attention on the present moment, accepting your thoughts and emotions without judgment, and letting go of negative thoughts and emotions. Research has shown that regular mindfulness meditation can reduce stress and anxiety, improve mood, and enhance emotional regulation.

2. Gratitude Practice

Cultivating a sense of gratitude can have a profound impact on our emotional well-being. It involves focusing on the positive aspects of our life and expressing gratitude for them. Gratitude practice can be as simple as keeping a gratitude journal or taking a few minutes each day to reflect on the things you are thankful for. Research has shown that gratitude practice can improve mood, increase resilience, and reduce stress.

3. Physical Exercise

Physical exercise is not only beneficial for our physical health but also for our emotional well-being. Exercise has been shown to reduce stress, anxiety, and depression, and enhance mood and self-esteem. It releases endorphins, which are natural mood-boosters, and promotes a sense of accomplishment and empowerment.

4. Self-Compassion Practice

Self-compassion involves treating ourselves with kindness, care, and understanding, especially during difficult times. It involves recognizing our common humanity and accepting ourselves as we are, with our flaws and imperfections. Self-compassion has been shown to reduce self-criticism, increase self-esteem and resilience, and improve emotional well-being.

5. Social Connection

Social connection is essential for our emotional well-being. It involves building and maintaining supportive relationships with others, such as friends, family, and community. Social connection provides us with a sense of belonging, support, and validation, and helps us cope with stress and adversity.

6. Relaxation Techniques

Relaxation techniques such as deep breathing, progressive muscle relaxation, and visualization can help reduce stress and promote emotional well-being. They involve slowing down and focusing on the present moment, letting go of negative thoughts and emotions, and promoting a sense of calm and relaxation.

7. Creative Expression

Engaging in creative activities such as art, music, or writing can be a powerful way to promote emotional well-being. Creative expression allows us to explore our thoughts and emotions, release pent-up emotions, and promote a sense of meaning and purpose. It can also enhance self-esteem and provide a sense of accomplishment and pride.

In conclusion, fostering inner peace and emotional well-being is essential for a fulfilling and meaningful life. By incorporating practices and strategies such as mindfulness meditation, gratitude practice, physical exercise, self-compassion, social connection, relaxation techniques, and creative expression, we can enhance our emotional well-being and live a more joyful and fulfilling life.

4.4.4 - Embracing the aging process with gratitude, acceptance, and grace

As we age, it's natural for our bodies and minds to change. These changes can sometimes be difficult to accept, and we may feel frustrated, anxious, or even depressed. However, by embracing the aging process with gratitude, acceptance, and grace, we can shift our perspective and find peace and contentment in the later years of our lives.

One way to embrace the aging process is to practice gratitude. Gratitude is a powerful tool that can help us focus on the positive aspects of our lives and cultivate feelings of contentment and happiness. We can cultivate gratitude by taking time each day to reflect on the things we are thankful for, whether it's our health, our relationships, or our experiences.

Acceptance is another key aspect of embracing the aging process. It's important to acknowledge that our bodies and minds will change as we age, and that this is a natural part of life. By accepting these changes, we can focus on the things that we can still do, rather than dwelling on the things that we may no longer be able to do.

Finally, embracing the aging process with grace means treating ourselves with kindness and compassion, and finding ways to enjoy life no matter what our age. This might involve exploring new hobbies, spending time with loved ones, or simply taking time each day to relax and enjoy the present moment.

In conclusion, by embracing the aging process with gratitude, acceptance, and grace, we can find fulfillment and contentment in our later years. We can shift our focus from what we may have lost to what we still have, and find joy in the simple pleasures of life.

Chapter 5: Planning for the Future: Financial Security and Legal Considerations

5.1: Financial Planning for Longevity

5.1.1 - The importance of financial planning and saving for retirement

Financial planning and saving for retirement are essential elements of a well-rounded and fulfilling life. Retirement is a time of life that should be enjoyed, not endured, and financial planning is the key to making this possible. It is important to start thinking about retirement planning as early as possible, even if you're still in your twenties or thirties.

One of the primary reasons for starting early is that the earlier you start, the more time you have to save and invest. Starting early also allows you to take advantage of compounding interest, which is the growth of your investments over time. The more time you have, the more your money can grow, and the greater your financial security in retirement.

Another reason for starting early is that you will have a clearer picture of your long-term financial goals. Setting goals for your retirement, such as the type of lifestyle you want to lead, the places you want to travel, and the activities you want to pursue, will help you determine how much money you need to save and invest to achieve those goals.

It is also important to have a plan in place for unexpected events that could impact your retirement savings, such as a medical emergency or job loss. Having an emergency fund and appropriate insurance coverage can help protect your retirement savings and ensure that you are prepared for any unexpected financial challenges.

In addition to saving and investing, it is important to develop good financial habits and make wise financial decisions throughout your life. This includes creating a budget, living within your means, and avoiding high-interest debt. It also means making smart investment choices and regularly reviewing and adjusting your investment portfolio as needed.

Retirement is a time of life that should be anticipated with excitement and optimism, and financial planning is a critical component of ensuring a secure and fulfilling retirement. By starting early, setting clear goals, developing good financial habits, and making wise investment choices, you can create a solid foundation for a successful retirement.

5.1.2 - Strategies for building a diverse and secure financial portfolio

Financial planning is an important part of ensuring lifelong stability and independence, especially as one approaches retirement age. Building a diverse and secure financial portfolio is key to achieving this goal, and requires a combination of thoughtful planning, sound investment strategies, and disciplined execution.

One key strategy for building a strong financial portfolio is diversification. This means spreading your investments across a range of asset classes, such as stocks, bonds, real estate, and commodities. By diversifying, you can help protect yourself against the risk of any one asset class declining in value, while also potentially increasing your returns over time.

Another important consideration is asset allocation. This refers to the process of determining how much of your portfolio should be invested in each asset class, based on your goals, risk tolerance, and time horizon. A common rule of thumb is to allocate a higher percentage of your portfolio to stocks when you are younger, and gradually shift towards bonds and other fixed-income investments as you approach retirement age.

In addition to diversification and asset allocation, it's also important to regularly review and rebalance your portfolio to ensure it remains aligned with your goals and risk tolerance. This may involve selling assets that have performed well and reinvesting the proceeds in other areas, or adjusting your asset allocation to reflect changes in your life circumstances or market conditions.

Another key strategy for building a secure financial portfolio is to focus on long-term growth rather than short-term gains. This means avoiding the temptation to chase hot stocks or other investments that may be volatile or speculative, and instead focusing on investing in quality companies or assets that have a track record of delivering solid returns over time.

Ultimately, building a diverse and secure financial portfolio requires discipline, patience, and a commitment to regularly reviewing and adjusting your strategy as needed. By working with a financial advisor or other qualified professional, you can develop a customized plan that meets your specific goals and helps ensure your long-term financial stability and independence.

5.1.3 - Navigating Social Security, pensions, and other retirement benefits

As retirement approaches, many people begin to think about the financial resources they will have available to them. Social Security, pensions, and other retirement benefits can provide a significant portion of the income retirees need to maintain their lifestyle. However, navigating the complex world of retirement benefits can be challenging. In this chapter, we will explore the key considerations related to Social Security, pensions, and other retirement benefits, and provide strategies for maximizing these resources.

Understanding Social Security

Social Security is a federal program that provides retirement, disability, and survivor benefits to eligible individuals. Eligibility for Social Security retirement benefits is based on the number of credits an individual has earned throughout their working life. Credits are earned by working and paying Social Security taxes, and the number of credits needed to qualify for retirement benefits varies based on an individual's birth year.

The amount of Social Security retirement benefits an individual will receive is based on their average earnings over their working life. The Social Security Administration calculates an individual's benefit amount using a formula that takes into account their highest 35 years of earnings. The amount of the benefit is also affected by the age at which an individual begins to receive benefits.

Strategies for Maximizing Social Security Benefits

One strategy for maximizing Social Security retirement benefits is to delay claiming benefits until age 70. For each year an individual delays claiming benefits beyond their full retirement age, the benefit amount increases by 8%. This can be a particularly effective strategy for individuals who have other sources of income to rely on during their early retirement years.

Another strategy for maximizing Social Security benefits is to coordinate benefits with a spouse. Spouses are entitled to a spousal benefit equal to 50% of their partner's benefit amount, provided they meet certain criteria. If both spouses have earned their own Social Security benefits, they may be able to claim one benefit first and then switch to the other later, in order to maximize their overall benefit amount.

Understanding Pensions

A pension is a retirement benefit that is paid out by an employer or a union. Pensions are typically based on an individual's salary and years of service, and the benefit amount is often determined by a formula set out in the pension plan.

Some pensions are also subject to cost-of-living adjustments (COLAs), which increase the benefit amount over time to account for inflation.

Strategies for Maximizing Pension Benefits

One strategy for maximizing pension benefits is to participate in a pension plan for as long as possible. This may mean staying with the same employer for many years or, for individuals who have changed jobs, consolidating pensions from multiple employers into a single plan.

Another strategy for maximizing pension benefits is to coordinate pension benefits with other sources of retirement income, such as Social Security or individual retirement accounts (IRAs). This can help ensure that retirees have a reliable and diverse stream of income throughout their retirement years.

Understanding Other Retirement Benefits

In addition to Social Security and pensions, there are many other retirement benefits that may be available to retirees. These may include benefits provided by a former employer or union, such as health insurance or life insurance, as well as benefits provided by government programs, such as Medicare or Medicaid.

Strategies for Maximizing Other Retirement Benefits

One strategy for maximizing other retirement benefits is to take advantage of all available benefits. This may require doing some research to identify the benefits that are available, and working with a financial advisor to develop a plan for maximizing those benefits.

Another strategy for maximizing other retirement benefits is to plan ahead for healthcare costs. Healthcare can be a significant expense for retirees, and understanding the options for Medicare, Medicaid, and other healthcare programs can help retirees make informed decisions about their healthcare coverage.

Conclusion

Navigating the complex world of retirement benefits can

5.1.4 - Budgeting, managing expenses, and creating a sustainable lifestyle

When it comes to retirement planning, it's not just about saving enough money. It's also about managing your expenses and creating a sustainable lifestyle that aligns with your financial goals. In this chapter, we'll explore the importance of budgeting, managing expenses, and creating a sustainable lifestyle in retirement planning.

Budgeting:

The first step in managing your expenses is creating a budget. A budget is a plan for how you will spend your money over a specific period. It can help you stay on track with your financial goals, prioritize your spending, and avoid overspending. When creating a budget, you should start by identifying your sources of income, such as Social Security, pensions, and investment income. You should also identify your fixed expenses, such as housing, insurance, and taxes, as well as your variable expenses, such as groceries, entertainment, and travel. Once you have a clear understanding of your income and expenses, you can develop a budget that balances your spending with your income and financial goals.

Managing Expenses:

In retirement, managing expenses is essential to ensure that you don't outlive your savings. One way to manage expenses is by cutting unnecessary costs. For example, you could reduce your cable bill, cancel subscriptions you don't use, or shop for cheaper groceries. You could also downsize your home, sell a car, or avoid eating out frequently. Additionally, you should be mindful of your spending habits and avoid overspending on non-essential items.

Creating a Sustainable Lifestyle:

Creating a sustainable lifestyle means living within your means and making choices that support your financial goals. This could include choosing to live in a less expensive area, driving an older car, or choosing a more modest lifestyle. By living sustainably, you can reduce your expenses and extend the life of your retirement savings.

Conclusion:

In retirement planning, budgeting, managing expenses, and creating a sustainable lifestyle are all important factors to consider. By creating a budget, managing your expenses, and making sustainable choices, you can ensure that you are living within your means and staying on track with your financial goals. Remember, retirement planning is a journey, and by taking these steps, you can make the most of it.

5.2: Estate Planning and Asset Protection

5.2.1 - The importance of estate planning for preserving your legacy

Estate planning is an essential part of financial planning and is critical to ensuring that your assets are distributed according to your wishes after you pass away. It is never too early to start estate planning, as it can help you ensure that your family and loved ones are taken care of in the event of your death.

One of the primary goals of estate planning is to avoid probate, which can be a lengthy and expensive process. Probate is the legal process that occurs after someone dies, and it involves determining the validity of the deceased person's will, paying off any debts, and distributing the remaining assets to the heirs.

There are several strategies that can be used to avoid probate, including creating a living trust, designating beneficiaries on retirement accounts and life insurance policies, and gifting assets during your lifetime. It is important to work with an experienced estate planning attorney to determine the best strategy for your particular situation.

In addition to avoiding probate, estate planning can also help minimize taxes and ensure that your assets are distributed according to your wishes. This may involve setting up a trust, creating a will, and designating guardians for minor children.

Another important aspect of estate planning is to ensure that you have the proper documents in place in the event that you become incapacitated or unable to make decisions for yourself. These documents may include a durable power of attorney, a health care directive, and a living will.

In summary, estate planning is a critical aspect of financial planning and is essential to ensuring that your assets are distributed according to your wishes. It is important to start estate planning early and work with an experienced attorney to develop a comprehensive plan that meets your needs and goals.

5.2.2 - Creating a will, trust, and other essential estate planning documents

Estate planning is a crucial aspect of financial planning and involves making decisions about how your assets will be distributed after you pass away. This process involves creating a will, trust, and other essential estate planning documents. A will is a legal document that outlines how your assets will be distributed after your death. A trust is a legal entity that holds assets for the benefit of a beneficiary.

Creating a will is an essential step in estate planning, as it ensures that your assets are distributed according to your wishes after your death. A will should be updated regularly to reflect any changes in your life, such as marriage, divorce, the birth of a child, or the purchase of new assets. It's important to choose an executor to manage your affairs after your death and to ensure that your wishes are carried out.

A trust is another important estate planning document that can help protect your assets and provide for your loved ones after your death. There are many different types of trusts, and the type that you choose will depend on your individual circumstances. For example, a revocable living trust allows you to retain control of your assets during your lifetime and ensures that they are distributed according to your wishes after your death.

In addition to a will and trust, there are several other essential estate planning documents that you should consider creating. These include a power of attorney, a health care directive, and a living will. A power of attorney allows you to designate someone to make financial decisions on your behalf if you become incapacitated. A health care directive and living will outline your wishes for medical treatment if you are unable to make decisions for yourself.

When creating estate planning documents, it's important to work with an experienced estate planning attorney who can help you navigate the legal complexities of the process. An attorney can ensure that your documents are legally binding and that they reflect your wishes. They can also provide guidance on strategies to minimize estate taxes and ensure that your assets are protected for future generations.

In conclusion, creating a will, trust, and other essential estate planning documents is a crucial aspect of financial planning. These documents can help ensure that your assets are distributed according to your wishes, protect your assets, and provide for your loved ones after your death. Working with an experienced estate planning attorney can help you navigate the legal complexities of the process and ensure that your wishes are carried out.

5.2.3 - Understanding tax implications and strategies for asset protection

When planning for the future, one of the most important considerations is how to protect and manage assets effectively. Estate planning is a critical component of this process, providing individuals with a framework for preserving their wealth and ensuring that their assets are distributed according to their wishes after they pass away. However, estate planning involves much more than simply creating a will, and requires a comprehensive understanding of the various tax implications and strategies for asset protection.

In this chapter, we will discuss the key elements of effective estate planning, including the importance of creating a will and other essential estate planning documents, understanding tax implications, and implementing strategies for asset protection.

Section 1: The Importance of Estate Planning for Preserving Your Legacy

Estate planning is a process that involves the preparation of legal documents to manage and distribute an individual's assets upon their death. It is a crucial step in protecting one's legacy and ensuring that their wishes are carried out after they pass away. Some of the key benefits of estate planning include:

1. Preserving your wealth and assets: Estate planning allows individuals to preserve their wealth and ensure that their assets are distributed according to their wishes after they pass away.

2. Protecting your family: Estate planning can provide financial security for loved ones, including children and other dependents, by ensuring that they are provided for in the event of one's death.

3. Minimizing taxes: Effective estate planning can help minimize tax liabilities, preserving more assets for future generations.

4. Avoiding probate: Estate planning can also help avoid probate, which can be a lengthy and expensive process that can tie up assets for months or even years.

Section 2: Creating a Will, Trust, and Other Essential Estate Planning Documents

Creating a will is an essential component of effective estate planning. A will is a legal document that outlines an individual's wishes regarding the distribution of their assets upon their death. In addition to a will, there are several other important estate planning documents that should be considered, including:

1. Living Trust: A living trust is a legal document that allows assets to be placed into a trust during an individual's lifetime, with provisions for distribution upon their death.

2. Power of Attorney: A power of attorney is a legal document that designates an individual to act as an agent or representative on behalf of another person.

3. Health Care Proxy: A health care proxy is a legal document that designates an individual to make medical decisions on behalf of another person in the event that they become unable to do so themselves.

4. Living Will: A living will is a legal document that outlines an individual's wishes regarding medical treatment in the event that they become unable to make decisions for themselves.

Section 3: Understanding Tax Implications and Strategies for Asset Protection

Effective estate planning requires a comprehensive understanding of the various tax implications and strategies for asset protection. Some key considerations include:

1. Estate Tax: Estate tax is a tax on the transfer of property upon an individual's death. Effective estate planning can help minimize estate tax liabilities.

2. Gift Tax: Gift tax is a tax on the transfer of property during an individual's lifetime. Effective estate planning can help minimize gift tax liabilities.

3. Charitable Giving: Charitable giving can be a powerful estate planning tool, allowing individuals to support causes that are important to them while also minimizing tax liabilities.

4. Life Insurance: Life insurance can be an effective tool for protecting assets and providing for loved ones after an individual's death.

Conclusion:

Effective estate planning is a critical component of planning for the future and protecting one's assets and legacy. By creating a will and other essential estate planning documents, understanding tax implications, and implementing strategies for asset protection, individuals can ensure that their wishes are carried out after they pass away, and their loved ones are provided for.

5.2.4 - Planning for potential long-term care and healthcare expenses

As we age, it's important to consider the potential need for long-term care and healthcare expenses. According to the U.S. Department of Health and Human Services, about 70% of people over the age of 65 will require some form of long-term care in their lifetime. Planning for these expenses can help alleviate financial stress and ensure that you receive the necessary care in your golden years.

1. Understanding Long-Term Care and Healthcare Expenses

Long-term care refers to a range of services that include medical and non-medical care for individuals who have chronic illnesses or disabilities. These services can be provided at home, in a nursing home, or in an assisted living facility.

Long-term care can be expensive and can quickly deplete retirement savings if not planned for properly.

Healthcare expenses also need to be considered when planning for retirement. Medicare provides some coverage for medical expenses, but it doesn't cover everything, and out-of-pocket costs can be significant. Additionally, as we age, we may require more frequent medical care, including prescription drugs and medical equipment, which can add to our overall healthcare costs.

2. Planning for Long-Term Care and Healthcare Expenses

One of the best ways to plan for long-term care and healthcare expenses is to invest in long-term care insurance. This type of insurance can help cover the costs of home healthcare, assisted living, and nursing home care. Policies can vary, so it's important to understand what is and isn't covered before purchasing a policy.

Another option is to set up a Health Savings Account (HSA) or Flexible Spending Account (FSA) to cover out-of-pocket medical expenses. Both of these accounts allow individuals to contribute pre-tax dollars to pay for medical expenses.

It's also important to consider how your retirement savings will be allocated to cover long-term care and healthcare expenses. Some individuals choose to designate a specific portion of their savings for these expenses, while others choose to purchase annuities to provide guaranteed income for healthcare expenses.

3. Talking to Family Members about Long-Term Care

Having conversations with family members about long-term care can be difficult, but it's important to do so to ensure everyone is on the same page. It's essential to discuss preferences for long-term care and how those costs will be covered. This can help alleviate financial stress and ensure that everyone is aware of the potential costs associated with long-term care.

4. Conclusion

Planning for long-term care and healthcare expenses is an essential part of retirement planning. Understanding the potential costs and investing in insurance or designated savings can help alleviate financial stress and ensure that you receive the care you need in your golden years. Having open conversations with family members about long-term care preferences and costs can also help ensure everyone is on the same page and prepared for the future.

5.3: Legal Considerations and Decision-Making

5.3.1 - The importance of advance directives and powers of attorney

As we age, it's important to consider the possibility that we may not always be able to make decisions for ourselves. In such situations, advance directives and powers of attorney can be invaluable tools for ensuring that our wishes are respected and that our best interests are protected.

An advance directive is a legal document that outlines your preferences for medical treatment in the event that you become incapacitated and are unable to communicate your wishes. This document can provide guidance to your family, loved ones, and medical professionals in making decisions about your care, including end-of-life care.

There are several types of advance directives, including living wills, medical powers of attorney, and do-not-resuscitate (DNR) orders. A living will allows you to specify the types of medical treatments you would or would not want in specific situations, such as if you were in a persistent vegetative state. A medical power of attorney, on the other hand, designates a person (known as an agent or surrogate) to make healthcare decisions on your behalf if you are unable to do so. A DNR order instructs healthcare providers not to perform cardiopulmonary resuscitation (CPR) in the event of cardiac or respiratory arrest.

It's important to discuss your wishes with your loved ones and healthcare providers and to ensure that your advance directives are up-to-date and legally binding. In some states, you may need to have your advance directives notarized or witnessed by a certain number of individuals.

In addition to advance directives, it's also important to consider appointing a power of attorney. A power of attorney is a legal document that designates a person (known as an attorney-in-fact or agent) to act on your behalf in financial or legal matters if you become incapacitated or are otherwise unable to manage your own affairs.

There are several types of powers of attorney, including durable powers of attorney, limited powers of attorney, and springing powers of attorney. A durable power of attorney grants your agent the authority to act on your behalf in financial or legal matters even if you become incapacitated. A limited power of attorney grants your agent limited authority to act on your behalf for a specific purpose and period of time. A springing power of attorney only takes effect if and when you become incapacitated.

When appointing a power of attorney, it's important to choose someone you trust and who is capable of handling your affairs in a responsible and ethical manner. You should also discuss your wishes and expectations with your agent and ensure that they are aware of their responsibilities and obligations.

In conclusion, advance directives and powers of attorney are important tools for ensuring that your wishes are respected and your best interests are protected in the event that you are unable to make decisions for yourself. By taking the time to discuss your wishes with your loved ones and healthcare providers and by appointing a trusted agent to act on your behalf, you can have peace of mind knowing that your affairs are in order and that your wishes will be honored.

5.3.2 - Understanding guardianship, conservatorship, and other legal protections

As we age, it becomes increasingly important to have legal protections in place to ensure our interests are safeguarded in the event of incapacity or disability. Two commonly used legal protections are guardianship and conservatorship. In this chapter, we will explore these legal protections and other options available to protect ourselves and our loved ones.

Guardianship:

A guardianship is a legal arrangement where a court appoints an individual or entity to care for a person who is unable to care for themselves. A guardian may be appointed for a minor child or for an adult who is incapacitated due to illness, disability, or injury.

Guardianship involves the transfer of legal authority from the person who is incapacitated to the appointed guardian. The guardian is responsible for making decisions related to the individual's personal care, such as housing, medical care, and education. The guardian is also responsible for managing the individual's finances, if necessary.

There are two types of guardianship: guardianship of the person and guardianship of the estate. Guardianship of the person is the appointment of a guardian to make personal care decisions for the incapacitated person. Guardianship of the estate is the appointment of a guardian to manage the individual's finances.

Conservatorship:

Conservatorship is another legal arrangement that involves the appointment of an individual or entity to manage the financial affairs of an incapacitated person. Unlike guardianship, conservatorship only involves the management of finances and does not involve the transfer of legal authority over the incapacitated person's personal care.

Conservatorship is often established when an individual has not created a durable power of attorney, which would allow a designated agent to manage their finances in the event of incapacity or disability. A conservatorship can be limited to a specific task, such as managing the sale of a property or it can be a more comprehensive arrangement that involves managing all aspects of the incapacitated person's finances.

Other legal protections:

In addition to guardianship and conservatorship, there are other legal protections available to protect ourselves and our loved ones. These include:

- Durable power of attorney: This is a legal document that allows an individual to designate an agent to manage their finances in the event of incapacity or disability. A durable power of attorney remains in effect even if the individual becomes incapacitated.

- Living will: A living will is a legal document that outlines an individual's wishes for medical care in the event they become incapacitated and are unable to make decisions for themselves.

- Health care proxy: A health care proxy is a legal document that designates an agent to make medical decisions for an individual who is unable to make decisions for themselves.

- Trusts: Trusts can be used to manage and protect assets and provide for loved ones in the event of incapacity or death.

Conclusion:

Legal protections such as guardianship, conservatorship, durable power of attorney, living wills, health care proxies, and trusts are all important tools that can be used to protect ourselves and our loved ones as we age. It is important to consult with an experienced attorney to determine which legal protections are appropriate for your specific situation.

5.3.3 - Planning for potential incapacity and end-of-life decisions

Planning for the end of one's life can be a difficult and emotionally challenging process, but it is an important aspect of overall financial planning. In addition to creating a will and establishing an estate plan, individuals should also consider planning for potential incapacity and end-of-life decisions. This includes creating advance directives and making decisions about medical treatment, as well as designating a trusted individual to make decisions on one's behalf if they become unable to do so themselves.

One of the most important aspects of planning for potential incapacity is creating advance directives. Advance directives are legal documents that allow individuals to specify their wishes for medical treatment in the event they become incapacitated and are unable to make decisions for themselves. There are several types of advance directives, including living wills, durable power of attorney for health care, and do-not-resuscitate orders.

A living will is a legal document that specifies an individual's preferences for medical treatment if they are unable to make decisions for themselves. This may include preferences regarding life-sustaining treatment, such as ventilators and feeding tubes, as well as pain management and other end-of-life care. Living wills are often used in conjunction with durable power of attorney for health care, which designates a trusted individual to make medical decisions on one's behalf if they become incapacitated.

In addition to advance directives, individuals should also consider designating a trusted individual as their health care proxy. This is someone who can make decisions about medical treatment on one's behalf if they become unable to do so themselves. It is important to choose someone who is trustworthy, reliable, and understands one's wishes for medical treatment.

In addition to planning for potential incapacity, individuals should also make decisions about end-of-life care. This may include decisions about whether to receive life-sustaining treatment, where to receive care, and other preferences regarding end-of-life care. It is important to have open and honest conversations with loved ones about these decisions and to document them in advance directives and other legal documents.

Overall, planning for potential incapacity and end-of-life decisions is an important aspect of overall financial planning.

By creating advance directives, designating a health care proxy, and making decisions about end-of-life care, individuals can ensure that their wishes for medical treatment and end-of-life care are respected and that their loved ones are prepared to make decisions on their behalf if necessary.

5.3.4 - Navigating the legal system and finding qualified professional assistance

Planning for the future can be overwhelming, especially when it comes to legal matters such as estate planning, wills, and trusts. Navigating the legal system and finding qualified professional assistance can make the process much smoother.

The legal system can be complex and difficult to navigate, especially for those who have never had any experience with it before. It is essential to have a basic understanding of the legal system, the laws that apply to your situation, and the legal process before proceeding with any legal matter.

There are many different legal professionals who can help you with your estate planning needs. Some of the most common legal professionals include estate planning attorneys, elder law attorneys, and financial planners. It is important to find a qualified professional who has experience working with clients in similar situations as yours.

When choosing a legal professional, it is important to consider their qualifications, experience, and reputation. Look for professionals who are licensed and certified in their respective fields, and who have a track record of success working with clients in similar situations.

One way to find a qualified legal professional is to ask for referrals from friends, family, or trusted advisors. You can also search online for local professionals or contact professional organizations, such as the National Academy of Elder Law Attorneys or the American Bar Association.

It is also important to understand the fees associated with legal services. Legal fees can vary widely depending on the complexity of the matter and the experience of the professional. Be sure to ask for a detailed fee schedule and understand what services are included in the fee.

In addition to finding a qualified legal professional, it is important to educate yourself on the legal process and stay informed throughout the process. Ask questions and seek clarification on any issues that are unclear. Be sure to keep all legal documents organized and accessible.

In summary, navigating the legal system and finding qualified professional assistance can be crucial in ensuring that your estate planning needs are met. Take the time to educate yourself on the legal process and find a qualified professional who can guide you through the process with confidence and peace of mind.

5.4: Building a Support Network for the Future

5.4.1 - Cultivating a network of trusted advisors and professionals

In today's complex world, planning for the future requires more than just one's own efforts. A strong network of trusted advisors and professionals is essential for anyone looking to achieve financial security and peace of mind. These individuals can provide valuable expertise and guidance in areas such as financial planning, estate planning, and legal matters, among others.

Building a network of trusted advisors and professionals is not a one-time event, but rather a lifelong process that requires ongoing effort and attention. The following are some tips for cultivating a strong network:

1. Identify your needs: The first step in building a network of trusted advisors and professionals is to identify your needs. Determine what areas you need assistance in and what kind of expertise you require.

2. Seek recommendations: Talk to friends, family members, and colleagues to see if they have any recommendations for professionals who can meet your needs. Online reviews and directories can also be useful resources for finding professionals in your area.

3. Conduct interviews: Once you have identified potential advisors and professionals, conduct interviews to assess their qualifications, experience, and communication skills. It is important to feel comfortable with your advisors and professionals, as you will be sharing personal and financial information with them.

4. Establish clear expectations: Once you have selected your advisors and professionals, it is important to establish clear expectations for communication, services, and fees. Make sure

to get everything in writing to avoid misunderstandings or surprises down the road.

5. Maintain regular contact: Building a strong network of trusted advisors and professionals requires ongoing communication and interaction. Schedule regular meetings and check-ins to stay up-to-date on your progress and make any necessary adjustments to your plan.

6. Continuously evaluate your network: As your needs and circumstances change over time, it is important to continuously evaluate your network of advisors and professionals. Make sure they are still meeting your needs and providing valuable expertise.

By following these tips, you can build a strong network of trusted advisors and professionals to help you navigate the complex world of financial planning and achieve your long-term goals. Remember, building a network is an ongoing process that requires continuous attention and effort.

5.4.2 - Establishing a support system of friends, family, and community members

As we age, it becomes increasingly important to have a support system in place. A strong support system can help us navigate the challenges that come with aging, such as health issues, loss of loved ones, and changes in our living situations. Our support system can also provide us with companionship, comfort, and a sense of belonging. In this chapter, we will discuss the importance of establishing a support system of friends, family, and community members, and provide tips for building and maintaining these relationships.

Importance of a Support System

Research has shown that having a strong support system can have a positive impact on our physical and emotional well-being. For example, studies have found that individuals with a strong support system have lower levels of stress and anxiety, and are less likely to develop depression and other mental health issues. Additionally, a support system can provide us with practical assistance when we need it, such as help with transportation, household tasks, or running errands.

Support systems are especially important for older adults, who may be at greater risk of isolation and loneliness. As we age, we may experience changes in our social networks due to retirement, relocation, or the loss of friends and family members. A support system can help fill these gaps and provide us with the social interaction and sense of purpose that we need to thrive.

Building a Support System

Building a support system of friends, family, and community members takes time and effort, but the benefits are well worth it. Here are some tips for building and maintaining these relationships:

1. Cultivate new relationships: Join clubs or groups that align with your interests, volunteer in your community, or take

classes at a local community center or college. These are great opportunities to meet new people and build new relationships.

2. Stay in touch with family: Make an effort to stay in touch with family members, even if you don't live close by. Regular phone calls, emails, or video chats can help maintain these relationships.

3. Connect with old friends: Reach out to old friends and acquaintances to reconnect and catch up. Social media can be a great tool for reconnecting with people from your past.

4. Be a good listener: Being a good listener is an important part of building and maintaining relationships. Listen attentively when others speak, and show interest and empathy in their lives.

5. Show appreciation: Show your appreciation for the people in your support system. Thank them for their help, and let them know how much they mean to you.

Maintaining a Support System

Once you have established a support system, it is important to maintain these relationships. Here are some tips for maintaining your support system:

1. Keep in touch: Stay in regular contact with the people in your support system. Schedule regular phone calls, visits, or activities to keep these relationships strong.

2. Be reliable: Be reliable and follow through on your commitments. This will help build trust and strengthen your relationships.

3. Ask for help when you need it: Don't be afraid to ask for help when you need it. Your support system is there to assist you, and asking for help when you need it is a sign of strength, not weakness.

4. Be flexible: Be open to new experiences and activities, and be willing to try new things with the people in your support system.

Conclusion

A support system of friends, family, and community members is essential for a fulfilling and meaningful life. Building and maintaining these relationships takes time and effort, but the benefits are well worth it. By cultivating new relationships, staying in touch with family and old friends, and being a good listener and showing appreciation, you can build a strong support system that will help you navigate the challenges

5.4.3 - Communicating your wishes and expectations to your loved ones

When planning for the future, it is essential to consider not only your own needs but also the needs of your loved ones. It's important to communicate your wishes and expectations to your family members and other important people in your life to ensure that they understand your desires and can respect them. Discussing sensitive topics such as end-of-life care and estate planning can be challenging, but having these conversations can help avoid misunderstandings and conflicts in the future.

Here are some strategies for communicating your wishes and expectations to your loved ones:

1. Start the conversation early: It is best to have these conversations before a crisis occurs. Starting the conversation early can help you avoid stress and emotional reactions.

2. Choose the right time and place: Choose a time and place where everyone is relaxed and not distracted. This will allow everyone to focus on the conversation and give it the attention it deserves.

3. Be honest and open: Be honest about your wishes and expectations. This includes your values, beliefs, and preferences. Be open to hearing the opinions and concerns of your loved ones as well.

4. Use clear and simple language: Use language that is clear and easy to understand. Avoid using technical jargon or confusing terms.

5. Create a plan: Work together to create a plan that reflects your wishes and expectations. This can include a living will, advance directives, or a family care plan.

6. Involve the right people: Involve the people who are important to you and who will be impacted by your decisions.

This includes family members, close friends, and healthcare providers.

7. Keep the conversation going: Regularly check in with your loved ones to make sure that everyone is on the same page. This can help avoid misunderstandings and ensure that everyone's needs are being met.

By following these strategies, you can communicate your wishes and expectations effectively and create a plan that reflects your values and beliefs. Remember that these conversations can be challenging, but they are important for ensuring that your loved ones understand your desires and can respect them.

5.4.4 - Embracing change and adapting your plans as life unfolds

As we go through life, change is inevitable. No matter how much we plan and prepare, unexpected events can occur that force us to adapt and adjust our plans. This is especially true when it comes to retirement planning and estate planning, where we are often dealing with long-term goals and unknown future circumstances.

Embracing change and being flexible in our plans is key to navigating these uncertainties. Here are some tips for adapting your plans as life unfolds:

1. Stay open-minded: One of the most important things you can do is to stay open-minded and flexible. Be willing to change your plans as circumstances change, and be open to new

opportunities that arise. Sometimes the unexpected can lead to new and exciting paths that you may not have considered otherwise.

2. Review and update your plans regularly: It's important to review and update your plans regularly, especially as you approach retirement and beyond. Keep track of any changes in your financial situation, health, and personal circumstances, and adjust your plans accordingly.

3. Seek professional advice: Working with a financial advisor, estate planning attorney, or other professional can help you navigate the complexities of planning for the future. These professionals can provide valuable guidance and advice, and can help you make informed decisions about your plans.

4. Have a contingency plan: It's important to have a contingency plan in place in case unexpected events occur. This might include having a backup retirement plan, an emergency fund, or a plan for long-term care.

5. Maintain a positive attitude: Finally, maintaining a positive attitude can help you navigate change and uncertainty. Embrace new opportunities and stay focused on your goals, even when the path forward is unclear.

In conclusion, change is inevitable, and being able to adapt and adjust our plans is key to navigating life's uncertainties. By staying open-minded, reviewing and updating our plans regularly, seeking professional advice, having a contingency plan, and maintaining a positive attitude, we can be better prepared to handle whatever life throws our way.

Chapter 6: The Future of Aging: Technological Innovations and Scientific Discoveries

6.1: Digital Health and Wearable Technologies

6.1.1 - The role of digital health in monitoring and managing personal health

The digital revolution has transformed almost every aspect of our lives, and the field of healthcare is no exception. Digital health, also known as eHealth or health technology, refers to the use of technology to improve health and healthcare. From wearable devices that monitor our physical activity and sleep patterns, to telemedicine platforms that connect patients with healthcare professionals remotely, digital health has the potential to revolutionize how we monitor and manage our personal health.

One of the key benefits of digital health is the ability to collect and analyze data about our health in real-time. Wearable devices such as smartwatches and fitness trackers can track everything from our heart rate and blood pressure to our sleep patterns and daily activity levels. This data can then be used to identify trends and patterns that may be indicative of underlying health issues, and to make more informed decisions about our lifestyle and healthcare choices.

Digital health also has the potential to improve access to healthcare, particularly for those living in remote or underserved areas. Telemedicine platforms allow patients to connect with healthcare professionals remotely, enabling them to receive diagnoses, prescriptions, and medical advice without having to travel long distances to a doctor's office or hospital. This can be particularly beneficial for those with chronic conditions that require ongoing monitoring and management.

However, digital health is not without its challenges. Privacy and security concerns around the collection and storage of personal health data must be carefully addressed to ensure that patients' rights are protected. There is also a risk that relying too heavily on technology may lead to a dehumanization of healthcare, with patients and healthcare professionals becoming disconnected from one another.

Despite these challenges, the potential benefits of digital health are significant. By embracing new technologies and digital tools, we can monitor and manage our personal health more effectively than ever before. From tracking our daily physical activity and sleep patterns, to connecting with healthcare professionals remotely, digital health has the potential to revolutionize how we approach our own health and wellbeing.

6.1.2 - Wearable technologies and their potential impact on longevity

As we enter the digital age, new innovations are being developed to improve our daily lives, including healthcare. One of the most significant developments in healthcare technology is the use of wearable technologies. These devices can help monitor and manage personal health, potentially leading to improved longevity.

Wearable technologies, such as smartwatches, fitness trackers, and health sensors, have become increasingly popular in recent years. These devices can monitor a range of biometric data, including heart rate, blood pressure, sleep patterns, and physical activity. This data can be analyzed and used to create personalized health plans, allowing individuals to make informed decisions about their health.

The potential impact of wearable technologies on longevity is significant. By tracking and analyzing personal health data, wearable technologies can provide early detection of health issues, leading to quicker diagnosis and treatment. This can potentially prevent the progression of chronic diseases and improve overall health outcomes.

Furthermore, wearable technologies can also encourage individuals to adopt healthier lifestyle habits, such as regular exercise and a balanced diet. By providing real-time feedback on physical activity and nutrition, these devices can help individuals set and achieve health goals, leading to improved longevity.

However, wearable technologies also pose some challenges. There are concerns about the accuracy and reliability of the data collected by these devices. Additionally, there is a risk of data breaches, leading to potential privacy concerns.

Overall, the potential benefits of wearable technologies on longevity are promising. With the development of more advanced technologies and improved data analysis, wearable technologies have the potential to revolutionize healthcare and improve longevity for individuals around the world.

6.1.3 - The future of personalized medicine and data-driven healthcare

The healthcare industry has always been a crucial aspect of human society, and with advancements in technology, it has become more personalized and data-driven than ever before. In this chapter, we will explore the future of personalized medicine and data-driven healthcare, how it is transforming the healthcare industry, and its potential impact on longevity.

Personalized Medicine:

Personalized medicine is a new approach to healthcare that focuses on the individual patient's unique genetic, environmental, and lifestyle factors. It is a shift from the traditional one-size-fits-all approach to healthcare, where patients receive the same treatment for a particular disease or condition. With personalized medicine, doctors can tailor treatments to individual patients based on their genetic makeup and other personal information.

Advancements in genetic testing and sequencing technologies have made personalized medicine a reality. Today, doctors can analyze a patient's DNA to identify genetic variations that may contribute to certain diseases or conditions. This information can be used to create personalized treatment plans that target the specific genetic factors contributing to the disease or condition.

Data-Driven Healthcare:

Data-driven healthcare is another aspect of the future of healthcare. It involves the collection, analysis, and use of patient data to improve healthcare outcomes. With the advancements in healthcare technology, healthcare providers can collect and analyze large amounts of patient data, including medical history, lifestyle, and environmental factors.

The data collected can be used to develop predictive models that can identify patients at risk of developing certain conditions, allowing doctors to take preventative measures before the disease progresses. Additionally, data-driven healthcare can help healthcare providers make better treatment decisions by providing them with real-time information on the patient's condition and response to treatment.

Impact on Longevity:

The future of personalized medicine and data-driven healthcare has the potential to significantly impact longevity. By tailoring treatments to individual patients, doctors can provide more effective and efficient treatments that may lead to better health outcomes. Additionally, the use of predictive models to identify patients at risk of developing certain conditions can allow doctors to take preventative measures, potentially reducing the risk of disease and increasing lifespan.

Moreover, the use of wearable technologies, such as fitness trackers and health monitors, can provide patients with real-time information on their health status, allowing them to take proactive measures to improve their health and prevent disease.

Conclusion:

The future of personalized medicine and data-driven healthcare is bright, with the potential to revolutionize the healthcare industry and impact longevity significantly. The use of genetic testing, predictive models, and wearable technologies can lead to more efficient and effective treatments, better disease prevention, and improved health outcomes. With continued advancements in technology, personalized medicine and data-driven healthcare will continue to transform the healthcare industry, paving the way for a healthier and longer life.

6.1.4 - Privacy, security, and ethical considerations in digital health

With the rise of digital health technologies, there is an increasing concern about privacy, security, and ethical considerations related to the use of personal health data. While these technologies have the potential to revolutionize healthcare by providing personalized and data-driven care, they also raise questions about who has access to this sensitive information and how it is being used.

Privacy Concerns in Digital Health

The use of digital health technologies generates a vast amount of personal health data, including medical history, biometric data, and behavioral data. This information can be used to create a detailed profile of an individual's health status and is therefore highly sensitive. As such, protecting the privacy of this data is paramount.

One of the biggest concerns about privacy in digital health is the potential for data breaches. Hackers could gain access to personal health information and use it for nefarious purposes such as identity theft or blackmail. Additionally, there is a risk that this data could be sold to third parties, such as insurance companies or employers, which could use it to make decisions about coverage or employment.

To address these concerns, regulations such as the Health Insurance Portability and Accountability Act (HIPAA) have been put in place to ensure that personal health information is protected. HIPAA requires healthcare providers to implement safeguards to protect patient data and to report any breaches that occur.

However, as digital health technologies continue to evolve, there may be a need for further regulations to ensure that privacy is protected. For example, there may need to be more strict regulations around the use of personal health data by third-party companies.

Security Concerns in Digital Health

In addition to privacy concerns, there are also security concerns related to digital health technologies. As more devices and systems are connected to the internet, there is an increased risk of cyberattacks.

These attacks could range from simple data breaches to more complex attacks, such as those that target medical devices themselves. For example, a hacker could gain access to a pacemaker and manipulate its settings, potentially causing harm to the patient.

To mitigate these risks, digital health technologies must be designed with security in mind from the outset. This means implementing strong authentication protocols, encryption, and other security measures to prevent unauthorized access.

Ethical Considerations in Digital Health

There are also ethical considerations related to the use of digital health technologies. One of the biggest concerns is the potential for these technologies to exacerbate existing health disparities. For example, individuals who do not have access to these technologies may not receive the same level of care as those who do.

Additionally, there is a concern that digital health technologies could be used to replace human interaction with healthcare providers. While these technologies can provide valuable insights into an individual's health, they cannot replace the empathy and care provided by a human healthcare provider.

Another ethical concern is the potential for these technologies to be used to discriminate against individuals based on their health status. For example, insurance companies could use personal health data to deny coverage or charge higher premiums.

To address these concerns, it is important that digital health technologies are designed with equity and inclusivity in mind. This means considering the needs of all individuals, including those who may not have access to these technologies.

Conclusion

Digital health technologies have the potential to revolutionize healthcare by providing personalized and data-driven care. However, they also raise important questions about privacy, security, and ethical considerations. To ensure that these technologies are used responsibly, it is important that regulations and standards are put in place to protect personal health data and to promote equity and inclusivity.

6.2: Virtual and Augmented Reality

6.2.1 - The potential of virtual and augmented reality in healthcare and wellness

Virtual and augmented reality (VR/AR) are innovative technologies that have shown immense potential in healthcare and wellness. In simple terms, VR involves the use of headsets and motion-tracking technology to simulate a virtual environment, while AR overlays digital information onto the real world. Both technologies offer new ways to interact with and understand health-related information, as well as improve overall wellbeing.

One of the primary applications of VR/AR in healthcare is pain management. Studies have shown that VR can help reduce pain by distracting patients and shifting their focus away from their discomfort. For example, VR experiences that take patients on a calming nature walk or a relaxing beach trip have been found to reduce pain and anxiety during medical procedures.

Another area where VR/AR shows potential is in mental health. By immersing patients in a virtual environment, therapists can expose them to anxiety-provoking situations in a controlled and safe way, allowing them to practice coping skills and gradually build resilience. AR also offers opportunities for enhancing mental health, such as providing real-time feedback on posture or breathing patterns to promote mindfulness and reduce stress.

VR/AR can also be used for training and education purposes. Medical professionals can use VR simulations to practice complex surgical procedures and emergency response scenarios in a risk-free environment. Additionally, AR can provide real-time information and guidance during medical procedures, such as overlaying 3D images of internal organs during surgery to help guide the surgeon's actions.

However, as with any new technology, there are ethical considerations to be aware of when it comes to VR/AR in healthcare. These include issues around privacy and data protection, as well as the potential for creating false memories or altering patients' perceptions of reality. It is important for healthcare professionals and researchers to approach the use of VR/AR with caution and to carefully consider the potential risks and benefits.

Overall, the potential applications of VR/AR in healthcare and wellness are vast and exciting. As the technology continues to evolve and become more accessible, we can expect to see more innovative uses and positive outcomes for patients and healthcare professionals alike.

6.2.2 - Enhancing cognitive stimulation and social engagement through immersive technologies

The advancements in technology have transformed our daily lives, from the way we communicate with each other to the way we work and learn. In recent years, virtual and augmented reality (VR/AR) technologies have emerged as an innovative tool to improve cognitive stimulation and social engagement among individuals of all ages.

Cognitive Stimulation through Immersive Technologies

One of the key benefits of immersive technologies is their ability to provide cognitive stimulation. This can be particularly beneficial for individuals who may be experiencing cognitive decline due to aging or other factors.

Research has shown that immersive technologies can help improve cognitive abilities such as attention, memory, and spatial awareness. For example, VR/AR-based memory games and puzzles have been shown to improve memory recall and attention span among older adults. Similarly, immersive technologies have been used to improve spatial navigation abilities among individuals with dementia.

In addition to improving cognitive abilities, immersive technologies can also enhance learning experiences. Virtual simulations can be used to provide hands-on training in a safe and controlled environment, which can be particularly useful in fields such as medicine and aviation.

Social Engagement through Immersive Technologies

Immersive technologies can also be used to promote social engagement, particularly among individuals who may be isolated or homebound due to physical or mental health conditions.

Virtual environments can provide a sense of social connectedness by allowing individuals to interact with others in a shared virtual space. This can be particularly beneficial for individuals who may have limited opportunities for social interaction in their daily lives.

Furthermore, VR/AR-based interventions have been shown to be effective in reducing social anxiety and improving social skills among individuals with autism spectrum disorders.

Considerations for the Use of Immersive Technologies

While immersive technologies offer great potential for cognitive stimulation and social engagement, it is important to consider certain ethical and practical considerations before their use.

Privacy and security are two key concerns when using immersive technologies, particularly when sensitive health information is involved. It is important to ensure that proper data security measures are in place to protect individuals' personal information.

Another consideration is accessibility, as not all individuals may have access to the necessary technology or may face physical or cognitive barriers to using immersive technologies.

Conclusion

Overall, immersive technologies offer promising opportunities to enhance cognitive stimulation and social engagement among individuals of all ages. With careful consideration of ethical and practical considerations, these technologies can be effectively used to improve quality of life and promote overall well-being.

6.2.3 - The role of virtual reality in pain management, rehabilitation, and mental health

Virtual Reality (VR) technology has come a long way since its inception in the 1980s. While it initially found use in gaming and entertainment industries, it has since been adopted in various fields, including healthcare. VR is a computer-generated environment that simulates a realistic sensory experience. It is designed to engage multiple senses, such as sight, sound, and touch, to create a feeling of presence and immersion in the virtual world.

In recent years, VR has been increasingly used in pain management, rehabilitation, and mental health treatment. Studies have shown that VR can effectively reduce pain, anxiety, and depression, enhance recovery after surgery or injury, and improve cognitive function.

Pain Management

Pain is a complex sensation that involves not only the physical experience but also emotional and psychological components. VR can help manage pain by distracting the patient from the pain sensation, reducing anxiety and stress, and promoting relaxation. VR is often used as a complementary therapy to traditional pain management techniques, such as medication and physical therapy.

Several studies have found that VR can effectively reduce pain in various conditions, such as acute and chronic pain, cancer-related pain, and procedural pain. For example, a study published in the Journal of Pain found that using VR during burn wound care procedures reduced pain intensity and distress in children.

Rehabilitation

VR can also be used in rehabilitation to help patients regain physical function after an injury or surgery. VR can provide a safe and controlled environment for patients to practice movements, build strength and endurance, and improve balance and coordination.

Studies have shown that VR-based rehabilitation can be effective in improving outcomes in various conditions, such as stroke, traumatic brain injury, and spinal cord injury. For example, a study published in the Journal of NeuroEngineering and Rehabilitation found that VR-based training improved arm function in stroke patients.

Mental Health

VR has also shown potential in the treatment of mental health conditions, such as anxiety disorders, post-traumatic stress disorder (PTSD), and phobias. VR-based therapies can provide a safe and controlled environment for patients to confront and overcome their fears and anxieties.

Studies have shown that VR-based therapies can be effective in reducing symptoms of various mental health conditions. For example, a study published in the Journal of Anxiety Disorders found that VR-based exposure therapy was effective in reducing symptoms of social anxiety disorder.

Privacy and Ethical Considerations

As with any technology, there are privacy and ethical considerations that must be addressed when using VR in healthcare. For example, VR-based therapies require the collection and storage of personal health information, which must be protected and secured. Patients must also be informed about the potential risks and benefits of VR-based therapies and must give their informed consent before participating.

In conclusion, VR has shown great promise in the field of healthcare, particularly in pain management, rehabilitation, and mental health treatment. As the technology continues to advance, it is likely that VR will become increasingly integrated into healthcare practices. However, it is essential that privacy and ethical considerations are addressed to ensure the safe and responsible use of VR in healthcare.

6.2.4 - The future of virtual and augmented reality in promoting healthy aging

Virtual and augmented reality (VR/AR) technologies have the potential to revolutionize the way we age by offering new ways to engage in physical and cognitive activities, promote social interaction, and manage health conditions. In this chapter, we will explore the ways in which VR/AR can be used to promote healthy aging, the challenges and opportunities of implementing these technologies, and the future of this field.

Promoting Physical Activity

One of the main benefits of VR/AR is its ability to provide engaging and interactive environments that can encourage physical activity in older adults. This is particularly important since physical activity is a key component of healthy aging, promoting muscle strength, balance, and flexibility, and reducing the risk of chronic conditions such as cardiovascular disease and diabetes.

Studies have shown that VR/AR can provide effective exercise programs that are more enjoyable and engaging than traditional methods. For example, VR/AR games can simulate activities such as dancing, cycling, or golfing, offering a more fun and interactive experience than traditional gym exercises. Moreover, VR/AR can be used to provide rehabilitation programs for seniors recovering from injuries or surgeries, offering a safe and controlled environment to practice movements and improve their mobility.

Promoting Cognitive Stimulation

VR/AR can also be used to promote cognitive stimulation, which is critical for maintaining brain health and reducing the risk of cognitive decline and dementia. Studies have shown that cognitive training programs using VR/AR can improve memory, attention, and executive function in older adults.

One example of a VR/AR program for cognitive stimulation is the use of "memory palaces." These are virtual environments that can be used to store and retrieve memories. By navigating a virtual environment and placing items in specific locations, seniors can practice their spatial memory and recall abilities.

Promoting Social Interaction

Social isolation is a common problem among older adults, leading to a range of physical and mental health issues. VR/AR can provide new opportunities for social interaction, offering virtual environments that can simulate real-life social situations.

For example, VR/AR can be used to connect seniors with family members and friends who live far away, offering a more immersive and engaging experience than traditional video calls.

Moreover, VR/AR can be used to create virtual communities and social events, allowing seniors to interact with others who share their interests and hobbies.

Challenges and Opportunities

Despite the potential benefits of VR/AR in promoting healthy aging, there are also several challenges that need to be addressed. One of the main challenges is the cost and accessibility of these technologies, particularly for seniors who may have limited financial resources or technological skills.

Another challenge is the need for tailored programs that are designed specifically for older adults. VR/AR programs need to take into account the physical, cognitive, and sensory changes that occur with aging, as well as the potential limitations and preferences of older users.

However, there are also several opportunities for promoting the adoption of VR/AR in aging populations. For example, VR/AR technologies can be integrated into existing healthcare systems, providing new ways to manage chronic conditions and reducing the need for in-person visits. Moreover, partnerships between technology companies, healthcare providers, and senior living communities can help to promote the development of tailored programs and the dissemination of these technologies.

Future Directions

The future of VR/AR in promoting healthy aging is promising, with ongoing research and development aimed at improving the accessibility, effectiveness, and acceptability of these technologies. For example, new VR/AR devices are being developed that are more affordable, user-friendly, and accessible to older adults.

Moreover, the integration of artificial intelligence (AI) and machine learning algorithms can help to personalize VR/AR programs to individual users' needs and preferences. AI can also be used

6.3: Robotics and Automation

6.3.1 - The role of robotics in supporting independent living and aging in place

As we age, we may face challenges in completing daily tasks, which can impact our ability to live independently. The use of robotics has emerged as a promising solution to support aging adults in their daily lives. Robotics can provide a range of benefits, including increased independence, improved safety, and enhanced quality of life.

In this chapter, we will explore the role of robotics in supporting independent living and aging in place. We will discuss the types of robotics that are available, their benefits, and the challenges associated with their use. We will also examine the future of robotics in aging care and its potential impact on society.

Types of Robotics for Aging Care

Robotic technology can be classified into four main categories: social robots, service robots, rehabilitation robots, and assistive robots. Each type has its unique set of functions, capabilities, and benefits for aging adults.

Social Robots

Social robots are designed to provide companionship and emotional support to aging adults. They can engage in conversations, play games, and even provide mental stimulation to prevent cognitive decline. Some examples of social robots include PARO, a robotic seal, and ElliQ, a social robot assistant.

Service Robots

Service robots are designed to help aging adults with daily tasks, such as cleaning, cooking, and grocery shopping. They can also monitor vital signs, remind patients to take their medication, and alert caregivers in case of an emergency. Some examples of service robots include the Roomba, a robotic vacuum cleaner, and the Cooki, a robotic kitchen assistant.

Rehabilitation Robots

Rehabilitation robots are designed to assist in the recovery process for aging adults who have suffered a stroke, injury, or disability. They can help with physical therapy, rehabilitation, and pain management. Some examples of rehabilitation robots include the Lokomat, a robotic gait training device, and the Hand of Hope, a robotic arm for stroke rehabilitation.

Assistive Robots

Assistive robots are designed to assist aging adults with mobility and transportation. They can help with tasks such as getting in and out of bed, standing up from a chair, and walking. Some examples of assistive robots include the HAL exoskeleton, a robotic suit that helps with mobility, and the AutoCrawler, a robotic wheelchair.

Benefits of Robotics for Aging Care

The use of robotics in aging care can provide numerous benefits to aging adults, their families, and society as a whole.

Increased Independence

Robotics can help aging adults maintain their independence by providing assistance with daily tasks. This can help them stay in their homes longer and avoid the need for institutional care.

Improved Safety

Robotics can also improve safety for aging adults by monitoring their health and well-being. For example, service robots can detect falls and alert caregivers, while rehabilitation robots can prevent injury during physical therapy.

Enhanced Quality of Life

Robotics can enhance the quality of life for aging adults by providing companionship, mental stimulation, and physical therapy. This can lead to improved mental health, cognitive function, and physical well-being.

Challenges of Robotics for Aging Care

Despite the numerous benefits of robotics for aging care, there are also several challenges that must be addressed.

Cost

Robotics can be expensive, which may limit their accessibility to aging adults who need them the most. This can be especially true for low-income individuals who may not have the financial resources to invest in this technology.

Privacy and Security

The use of robotics in aging care also raises concerns about privacy and security. For example, social robots may record conversations, which could compromise privacy. There is also the risk of hackers gaining access to personal health information, which could compromise security.

Acceptance and Adoption

The acceptance and adoption of robotics in aging care may also be

6.3.2 - The potential of robotic companions and caregivers in promoting emotional well-being

As people age, they may experience social isolation, loneliness, and a lack of companionship, which can lead to depression, anxiety, and other negative health outcomes. Robotic companions and caregivers have the potential to address these issues and promote emotional well-being among older adults.

Robotic companions are designed to provide emotional support, entertainment, and companionship to older adults. They can engage in conversation, play games, and provide reminders for medication and appointments. Some robotic companions also have the ability to learn and adapt to a person's preferences and habits, making them more personalized and engaging.

Robotic caregivers, on the other hand, are designed to assist with activities of daily living such as bathing, dressing, and meal preparation. They can also monitor vital signs and provide reminders for medication and appointments. Robotic caregivers have the potential to reduce the need for human caregivers and increase independence and autonomy among older adults.

While the potential benefits of robotic companions and caregivers are clear, there are also potential drawbacks and ethical considerations to consider. For example, some may argue that robotic companions and caregivers may contribute to further social isolation and a lack of human connection. Others may be concerned about the privacy and security of personal data collected by these devices.

To address these concerns, it is important to ensure that the development and use of robotic companions and caregivers are guided by ethical principles and regulatory frameworks. It is also important to involve older adults in the design and development process to ensure that these devices are user-friendly and meet their needs and preferences.

In conclusion, robotic companions and caregivers have the potential to promote emotional well-being and increase independence among older adults. However, it is important to consider potential drawbacks and ethical considerations and to ensure that these devices are developed and used in an ethical and responsible manner.

6.3.3 - The impact of automation on healthcare delivery and services

Automation is changing the healthcare industry in many ways, from improving patient care to streamlining administrative tasks. It has the potential to revolutionize healthcare delivery and services in a number of ways, but it also poses challenges that must be addressed.

One of the biggest advantages of automation in healthcare is the ability to improve patient outcomes. For example, automated systems can monitor patient vital signs and alert healthcare providers to potential problems, allowing for faster interventions and more effective treatments. Automated medication dispensing systems can also reduce the risk of medication errors, which can have serious consequences for patients.

Another area where automation can improve healthcare delivery is in administrative tasks. Automating tasks such as appointment scheduling, billing, and insurance claims processing can reduce errors and free up staff to focus on more complex tasks, such as patient care.

However, automation also poses challenges for healthcare providers. One of the biggest challenges is ensuring the accuracy and security of patient data. With more data being generated and stored electronically, there is a greater risk of data breaches and cyberattacks. Healthcare providers must implement robust security measures to protect patient data and ensure that automated systems are properly integrated with existing systems.

Another challenge is ensuring that automation is used appropriately and does not replace the human touch in healthcare. While automation can improve efficiency and accuracy, it cannot replace the compassion and empathy that human caregivers provide. Healthcare providers must strike a balance between using automation to improve care and ensuring that patients receive the human touch they need.

In addition, automation can also lead to job displacement for healthcare workers, particularly in administrative roles. As automation takes over routine tasks, healthcare workers will need to be retrained to take on more complex roles that cannot be automated.

Overall, the impact of automation on healthcare delivery and services is complex and multifaceted. While automation has the potential to improve patient outcomes and streamline administrative tasks, it also poses challenges that must be addressed. Healthcare providers must carefully consider the use of automation and ensure that it is used appropriately and responsibly.

6.3.4 - Ethical considerations and the future of human-robot interactions

As technology advances and robots become more integrated into our daily lives, it is important to consider the ethical implications of these developments, particularly in the context of healthcare and aging. While robots and automation have the potential to improve quality of life for older adults, there are also concerns about privacy, safety, and the impact on human relationships.

One ethical issue is the potential for robots to replace human caregivers and healthcare providers. While robots can assist with physical tasks and monitoring, they cannot provide the same level of emotional support and personal connection that human caregivers can offer. The use of robots in healthcare may also lead to job loss and a reduction in the number of human caregivers, which could negatively impact the quality of care provided to older adults.

Another ethical consideration is privacy and data security. Robots and other digital technologies collect and store vast amounts of personal data, which could be vulnerable to cyberattacks and misuse. There is a need for regulations and standards to protect the privacy and security of older adults who use these technologies.

Additionally, there are concerns about the potential for robots to perpetuate ageism and discrimination. If robots are designed and programmed to have biases against older adults, this could further marginalize and disadvantage this population. It is important to consider diversity and inclusion in the development and implementation of these technologies.

As human-robot interactions become more common, it is important to ensure that older adults have agency and control over their interactions with robots. This includes the ability to make informed decisions about their use of these technologies, as well as the ability to set boundaries and express their preferences.

In conclusion, the integration of robots and automation in healthcare and aging presents both opportunities and challenges. It is important to consider the ethical implications of these developments and to prioritize the well-being and agency of older adults. By doing so, we can ensure that these technologies are used in ways that promote independence, quality of life, and dignity for older adults.

6.4: Personalized Genomics and Precision Medicine

6.4.1 - The potential of personalized genomics in preventing and treating age-related diseases

As the field of genomics continues to evolve, personalized genomics is increasingly being used to better understand the genetic basis of age-related diseases and to develop more targeted prevention and treatment strategies. Personalized genomics involves analyzing an individual's genetic makeup to identify specific genetic variants or mutations that may increase their risk of developing certain diseases, such as cancer, Alzheimer's disease, or heart disease.

One of the key benefits of personalized genomics is that it can help individuals make more informed decisions about their health and lifestyle choices. For example, if someone learns they have a genetic predisposition to heart disease, they may be more motivated to adopt a healthier diet and exercise regimen to reduce their risk.

Another important application of personalized genomics is in the development of targeted therapies for specific diseases. By identifying the genetic mutations that are driving a particular disease, researchers can develop drugs that specifically target those mutations, potentially leading to more effective treatments with fewer side effects.

However, there are also important ethical and privacy considerations to be aware of when it comes to personalized genomics. For example, there is the risk that genetic information could be used to discriminate against individuals in areas such as employment or insurance coverage. Additionally, there is a need to ensure that genetic data is kept confidential and secure, to prevent it from being accessed by unauthorized individuals or entities.

Despite these challenges, the potential of personalized genomics to transform the way we prevent and treat age-related diseases is enormous. As this field continues to advance, it is likely to play an increasingly important role in promoting healthy aging and improving overall health outcomes for individuals.

6.4.2 - The role of precision medicine in tailoring healthcare to individual needs

Precision medicine, also known as personalized medicine, is an innovative approach to healthcare that tailors treatment plans to the unique genetic, environmental, and lifestyle factors of each patient. This approach recognizes that every individual is unique, and no two people respond to treatment the same way. Precision medicine takes a more targeted approach to care, aiming to maximize effectiveness while minimizing side effects.

The goal of precision medicine is to provide the right treatment, to the right person, at the right time. To achieve this goal, precision medicine relies on advanced technologies such as genomic sequencing, which allows for a more detailed understanding of an individual's genetic makeup. By analyzing a patient's genetic information, healthcare providers can identify specific mutations that may be causing a disease, predict how the patient is likely to respond to different treatments, and identify potential side effects.

Precision medicine has already been successful in treating a number of different diseases, including cancer, cardiovascular disease, and rare genetic disorders. For example, in cancer treatment, precision medicine has led to the development of targeted therapies that block specific genetic mutations driving tumor growth, resulting in better outcomes and fewer side effects.

In addition to genomic sequencing, precision medicine also involves the use of other technologies, such as wearable devices and electronic health records, to collect and analyze data about patients in real-time. This allows healthcare providers to monitor patients more closely and make more informed treatment decisions.

Precision medicine also has the potential to reduce healthcare costs by avoiding unnecessary treatments and minimizing side effects. By identifying the most effective treatment plan for each patient, precision medicine can reduce the need for expensive trial-and-error treatments that may not be effective.

However, there are challenges to implementing precision medicine on a large scale. The high cost of genomic sequencing and other technologies can make it difficult for many patients to access precision medicine. Additionally, there are concerns about the privacy and security of patient data, as well as the potential for genetic discrimination by insurance companies and employers.

Despite these challenges, precision medicine has the potential to revolutionize healthcare and improve patient outcomes. As technology continues to advance and become more affordable, precision medicine is likely to become more widely available and accessible, allowing healthcare providers to provide truly personalized care to patients.

6.4.3 - The future of genetic testing and personalized interventions

Advances in genetics and genomics have opened up new possibilities for personalized healthcare. Genetic testing has become increasingly accessible and affordable, enabling individuals to learn about their genetic makeup and potential health risks. With this information, healthcare providers can tailor interventions to a patient's specific genetic profile, potentially leading to more effective and targeted treatments.

The field of pharmacogenomics, which studies the relationship between a patient's genetics and their response to medication, is one area where personalized interventions are already being used. By analyzing a patient's genetic makeup, healthcare providers can identify potential adverse reactions to certain medications or predict which medications will be most effective for a particular individual. This approach can improve treatment outcomes while reducing the risk of harmful side effects.

Another area where genetic testing is being used for personalized interventions is in the field of cancer treatment. By analyzing the genetic mutations present in a patient's cancer cells, healthcare providers can identify the most appropriate treatment options for that individual. This approach, known as precision oncology, has led to more effective and targeted cancer treatments, improving survival rates and reducing the side effects of treatment.

As genetic testing becomes more sophisticated, there is potential for even more personalized interventions. For example, researchers are exploring the use of gene editing technologies such as CRISPR to correct genetic mutations that lead to disease. While still in the early stages of development, this approach has the potential to prevent or cure genetic diseases by editing the patient's DNA.

However, the use of genetic testing for personalized interventions raises ethical considerations around issues such as privacy and discrimination. Patients must have control over their genetic information and be able to make informed decisions about how it is used. Healthcare providers and researchers must also ensure that the use of genetic information does not lead to discrimination or stigmatization of individuals based on their genetic makeup.

In conclusion, the future of genetic testing and personalized interventions holds great promise for improving healthcare outcomes. As technology advances and our understanding of genetics and genomics grows, personalized interventions will become more sophisticated and targeted, leading to better health outcomes for individuals. However, it is important to ensure that ethical considerations are taken into account to protect patient privacy and prevent discrimination.

6.4.4 - Ethical, legal, and social implications of personalized genomics and precision medicine

As personalized genomics and precision medicine become more prevalent, there are many ethical, legal, and social implications to consider. While these fields offer immense potential for improving healthcare, they also raise important questions about privacy, equity, and access. In this chapter, we will explore some of the key ethical, legal, and social issues surrounding personalized genomics and precision medicine.

1. Privacy Concerns

Personalized genomics and precision medicine require the collection and analysis of large amounts of personal health information. This raises important questions about privacy and data security. Patients need to be assured that their genetic information and health data are being handled responsibly, and that their information is not being shared without their consent. Additionally, it is important to consider the possibility of discrimination based on genetic information, such as by employers or insurance companies. To address these concerns, there are laws and regulations in place to protect patient privacy, such as the Health Insurance Portability and Accountability Act (HIPAA) in the United States.

2. Equity and Access

One of the biggest challenges with personalized genomics and precision medicine is ensuring that everyone has access to these advances, regardless of their income or background. There are concerns that personalized genomics and precision medicine could further widen health disparities if only certain groups of people have access to these tools. It is important to consider how to make personalized genomics and precision medicine more affordable and accessible for everyone, and to ensure that these technologies are not only available to those who can afford to pay for them.

3. Informed Consent

Patients need to be fully informed about the potential benefits and risks of personalized genomics and precision medicine before they can make informed decisions about participating in these programs. This requires clear communication between patients and healthcare providers, as well as a comprehensive understanding of the technology and its implications. Informed consent should also include information about the potential for incidental findings – genetic information that may reveal unexpected health risks – and how this information will be handled.

4. Regulatory Oversight

Personalized genomics and precision medicine are relatively new fields, and there is a need for appropriate regulatory oversight to ensure that these technologies are being used safely and effectively. This includes ensuring that genetic testing is accurate and reliable, and that healthcare providers are using the results of these tests appropriately. Additionally, there is a need for ongoing research to understand the long-term implications of personalized genomics and precision medicine, and to ensure that these technologies are being used in ways that are ethical and socially responsible.

5. Societal Implications

Finally, personalized genomics and precision medicine have broader societal implications that need to be considered. For example, these technologies could lead to a greater focus on individual health and wellness, rather than on public health concerns. Additionally, there are concerns that personalized genomics and precision medicine could lead to increased medicalization of everyday life, as people become more focused on monitoring their health and seeking medical interventions. It is important to consider these broader implications as personalized genomics and precision medicine continue to evolve.

Conclusion:

Personalized genomics and precision medicine offer immense potential for improving healthcare and extending lifespan. However, these fields also raise important ethical, legal, and social concerns that need to be addressed. To ensure that personalized genomics and precision medicine are used safely, effectively, and responsibly, it is important to consider issues such as privacy, equity, access, informed consent, regulatory oversight, and societal implications. By addressing these concerns, we can help to ensure that personalized genomics and precision medicine are used to their full potential, while minimizing the risks and potential harms associated with these advances.

Chapter 7: Embracing the Journey: A Roadmap to a Fulfilling, Ageless Odyssey

7.1: Integrating Longevity Strategies into Daily Life

7.1.1 - Creating a personalized longevity plan: Assessing your needs and goals

In order to live a long and healthy life, it is important to create a personalized longevity plan. Such a plan should take into account your specific needs, goals, and current health status. In this chapter, we will discuss how to assess these factors and create a plan that is tailored to your individual needs.

The first step in creating a longevity plan is to assess your current health status. This may involve visiting your healthcare provider for a physical exam and lab tests to assess your cholesterol levels, blood pressure, and other key health indicators. It is important to know your current health status in order to identify any areas that may require attention.

Once you have assessed your current health status, you can begin to identify your goals for living a long and healthy life. This may include goals related to exercise, diet, stress management, and sleep. It is important to set specific, measurable goals that are achievable and realistic. For example, if you want to improve your fitness level, you might set a goal to walk for 30 minutes every day.

In addition to setting goals, it is important to identify the strategies that you will use to achieve those goals. This may include developing an exercise plan, creating a healthy eating plan, and practicing stress reduction techniques such as meditation or yoga.

Your longevity plan should also take into account any health conditions or risks that you may have. For example, if you have a family history of heart disease, your plan may include strategies to reduce your risk of developing this condition. It is important to work with your healthcare provider to develop a plan that is tailored to your individual needs.

Finally, your longevity plan should be flexible and adaptable. Life is unpredictable, and it is important to be able to adjust your plan as needed. Your plan should also take into account any changes in your health status or personal circumstances.

In summary, creating a personalized longevity plan involves assessing your current health status, setting goals, identifying strategies to achieve those goals, taking into account any health conditions or risks, and creating a flexible and adaptable plan. By taking these steps, you can increase your chances of living a long and healthy life.

7.1.2 - Implementing lifestyle changes and building healthy habits

In recent years, there has been a growing interest in lifestyle factors that can promote longevity and healthy aging. Many individuals are looking to implement changes in their daily routine to improve their health and quality of life. This chapter will explore some of the lifestyle changes and habits that can help support healthy aging.

The first step in creating a personalized longevity plan is to assess your needs and goals. This involves taking a comprehensive look at your current health status and identifying areas that may need improvement. You may want to consider consulting with a healthcare provider or other qualified professional to help you evaluate your current health and develop a plan for achieving your goals.

Once you have identified your needs and goals, the next step is to implement lifestyle changes and build healthy habits. Here are some suggestions for areas to focus on:

1. Exercise and physical activity: Regular exercise has been shown to have numerous health benefits, including reducing the risk of chronic diseases and improving mental health. Aim for at least 150 minutes of moderate-intensity exercise per week, or 75 minutes of vigorous-intensity exercise. Incorporating strength training and balance exercises can also be beneficial.

2. Nutrition: A balanced and nutritious diet is important for maintaining health and preventing chronic diseases. Aim to consume a variety of fruits, vegetables, whole grains, lean proteins, and healthy fats. Limit your intake of processed and high-fat foods, as well as sugary beverages.

3. Sleep: Adequate sleep is essential for overall health and well-being. Aim for 7-8 hours of sleep per night, and establish a consistent sleep schedule.

4. Stress management: Chronic stress can have negative effects on health and longevity. Implementing stress management techniques such as mindfulness meditation, deep breathing, and yoga can be beneficial.

5. Social connections: Maintaining social connections and engaging in meaningful activities can contribute to overall health and well-being. Consider joining a social group, volunteering, or participating in hobbies or interests that you enjoy.

6. Mental stimulation: Keeping the mind active and engaged is important for maintaining cognitive function and preventing age-related cognitive decline. Engage in mentally stimulating activities such as reading, puzzles, or learning a new skill.

7. Avoidance of harmful substances: Limiting or avoiding harmful substances such as tobacco, excessive alcohol, and illicit drugs is important for maintaining health and longevity.

By implementing these lifestyle changes and building healthy habits, individuals can support healthy aging and improve their overall quality of life. It is important to remember that every individual is unique, and a personalized approach is necessary to achieve optimal health and longevity. Working with a healthcare provider or other qualified professional can help ensure that your longevity plan is tailored to your individual needs and goals.

7.1.3 - Overcoming obstacles and maintaining motivation on your ageless journey

As you embark on your journey towards longevity, it's important to recognize that there will be obstacles and challenges along the way. Whether it's a lack of motivation, a busy schedule, or unexpected setbacks, it's important to have strategies in place to overcome these obstacles and stay on track. In this chapter, we'll explore some common obstacles to living a long and healthy life, as well as tips and strategies for maintaining motivation and overcoming challenges.

Identifying Your Obstacles

Before you can start developing strategies for overcoming obstacles, it's important to identify what those obstacles are. Everyone faces different challenges on their journey towards longevity, but some common obstacles include:

1. Lack of motivation: It can be difficult to stay motivated over the long term, especially if you're not seeing immediate results.

2. Busy schedule: Many people struggle to find time to prioritize their health and wellness amidst the demands of work, family, and other obligations.

3. Financial constraints: Some people may feel like they can't afford to prioritize their health and wellness, especially if healthy food and other resources are expensive.

4. Chronic health conditions: People with chronic health conditions may face additional challenges in maintaining their health and preventing further complications.

5. Social isolation: Social isolation and loneliness can have negative effects on mental and physical health, and can be a barrier to maintaining healthy habits.

Developing Strategies for Overcoming Obstacles

Once you've identified your obstacles, you can start developing strategies for overcoming them. Here are some tips and strategies that can help:

1. Set realistic goals: Instead of trying to make big changes all at once, focus on small, achievable goals that will help you make progress over time.

2. Find an accountability partner: Having someone to hold you accountable and provide support can be incredibly helpful in maintaining motivation and overcoming challenges.

3. Prioritize self-care: Make time for self-care activities that help you de-stress and recharge, such as exercise, meditation, or hobbies.

4. Seek out resources: There are many resources available that can help you overcome specific obstacles, whether it's financial assistance for healthy food, support groups for chronic health conditions, or social events that help combat social isolation.

5. Focus on the positive: Instead of dwelling on setbacks or negative experiences, focus on the positive changes you're making and celebrate your progress along the way.

Conclusion

Living a long and healthy life requires dedication and perseverance, but it's important to remember that you don't have to do it alone. By identifying your obstacles, developing strategies for overcoming them, and staying motivated and positive along the way, you can achieve your goals and enjoy the benefits of a long and fulfilling life.

7.1.4 - Continuously evaluating and refining your strategies for optimal well-being

In order to maintain optimal health and longevity, it is important to continuously evaluate and refine your strategies for well-being. This means assessing the effectiveness of your current lifestyle habits and making adjustments as necessary to achieve your goals.

One way to evaluate your strategies is to regularly track your progress. This can involve keeping a journal or using an app to monitor your physical activity, diet, sleep, and stress levels. By tracking your behaviors, you can identify patterns and trends, and make informed decisions about how to adjust your habits for better health.

It is also important to stay up-to-date on the latest research and recommendations related to healthy aging. New studies and discoveries are constantly emerging, and it is important to stay informed about the latest findings in order to make the best decisions for your health.

In addition to monitoring your behaviors and staying informed, it is also helpful to seek support and feedback from others. This can involve talking to friends, family members, or healthcare professionals about your goals and progress, and seeking their input on how to improve your strategies.

Finally, it is important to remain flexible and adaptable in your approach to healthy aging. As you age, your body and circumstances may change, and it is important to adjust your strategies accordingly. This may involve trying new activities or habits, seeking out new sources of support, or making modifications to your existing routines.

By continuously evaluating and refining your strategies for well-being, you can optimize your health and longevity, and enjoy a fulfilling and ageless life.

7.2: Building a Resilient Mindset

7.2.1 - The power of belief and mindset in shaping your aging experience

How you perceive aging, and your beliefs about it, can impact your aging experience. Positive beliefs about aging have been associated with better physical health, cognitive functioning, and mental well-being. In contrast, negative beliefs about aging can contribute to worse health outcomes, cognitive decline, and depression. In this chapter, we explore the power of belief and mindset in shaping your aging experience and offer strategies to cultivate a positive aging mindset.

The Impact of Beliefs and Mindset on Aging:

Your beliefs about aging can impact your physical and cognitive functioning. For instance, studies have shown that individuals who hold positive beliefs about aging have better physical health outcomes. They have better cardiovascular health, better balance, and walk faster than those with negative beliefs. Additionally, holding negative beliefs about aging can have harmful effects on cognitive function. Older adults who believe that aging leads to mental decline perform worse on cognitive tests than those with positive beliefs about aging.

Moreover, beliefs about aging can impact emotional well-being. Older adults with positive beliefs about aging report feeling happier, more satisfied with life, and more optimistic about their future. On the other hand, negative beliefs about aging have been associated with increased anxiety, stress, and depression.

Strategies to Cultivate a Positive Aging Mindset:

Fortunately, it is possible to cultivate a positive aging mindset. Here are some strategies that can help:

1. Challenge negative stereotypes about aging: Many negative stereotypes exist about aging, such as the belief that older adults are frail, forgetful, and lonely. By challenging these stereotypes, you can begin to see aging in a more positive light.

2. Engage in physical activity: Physical activity can have a positive impact on your physical and mental health. It can improve your balance, reduce the risk of chronic diseases, and boost mood.

3. Practice mindfulness: Mindfulness can help you cultivate a greater sense of well-being by focusing on the present moment and reducing stress and anxiety.

4. Engage in social activities: Social isolation can contribute to negative beliefs about aging. Engaging in social activities can help you stay connected to others and feel more positive about aging.

5. Develop a sense of purpose: Having a sense of purpose can provide meaning and direction in life, which can help you stay positive and motivated.

Conclusion:

Your beliefs about aging can impact your aging experience. By cultivating a positive aging mindset, you can improve your physical and mental well-being, and enjoy a more fulfilling life. By challenging negative stereotypes about aging, engaging in physical activity, practicing mindfulness, engaging in social activities, and developing a sense of purpose, you can create a positive aging experience for yourself.

7.2.2 - Cultivating resilience, adaptability, and a positive attitude

As we age, we are likely to experience a wide range of changes and challenges that can test our resilience and ability to adapt. These can include physical, cognitive, and emotional changes, as well as changes in our social and environmental circumstances. However, it is important to remember that our ability to adapt and bounce back from these challenges is not predetermined. It is a skill that can be developed and strengthened over time. In this chapter, we will explore the importance of cultivating resilience, adaptability, and a positive attitude, and provide practical tips for doing so.

Resilience:

Resilience is the ability to bounce back from adversity and maintain a sense of well-being in the face of stress or challenge. Resilient individuals are better equipped to cope with stress, overcome obstacles, and maintain a positive outlook on life. Here are some tips for cultivating resilience:

1. Practice self-care: Taking care of your physical, emotional, and spiritual needs can help you build the resilience you need to face life's challenges. Get enough sleep, eat well, exercise regularly, and take time for activities that bring you joy and fulfillment.

2. Build a support network: Having a strong network of family, friends, and community members can provide emotional support and help you cope with stress.

3. Develop problem-solving skills: Being able to identify problems and find solutions can help you feel more in control and better equipped to handle challenges.

4. Practice mindfulness: Mindfulness practices such as meditation, deep breathing, and yoga can help you develop a sense of calm and inner peace, even in the midst of stress.

Adaptability:

Adaptability is the ability to adjust to changing circumstances and remain flexible in the face of uncertainty. As we age, it is important to remain open to new experiences and opportunities, and to be willing to try new things. Here are some tips for cultivating adaptability:

1. Stay curious: Learning new things and exploring new experiences can help keep your mind active and engaged, and foster a sense of curiosity and wonder.

2. Embrace change: Change is a natural part of life, and being able to adapt to changing circumstances can help you maintain a sense of control and balance.

3. Be open-minded: Being willing to consider new ideas and perspectives can help you expand your horizons and find new solutions to problems.

4. Take risks: Trying new things and taking risks can help you build confidence and resilience, and can lead to new opportunities and experiences.

Positive Attitude:

Maintaining a positive attitude is important for overall well-being and can help you cope with stress and adversity. Here are some tips for cultivating a positive attitude:

1. Practice gratitude: Focusing on the things you are grateful for can help shift your perspective and promote a sense of positivity and well-being.

2. Surround yourself with positive people: Being around positive, supportive people can help lift your spirits and promote a sense of optimism.

3. Focus on the present moment: Mindfulness practices such as meditation can help you stay present and focused on the present moment, which can help reduce stress and promote a sense of calm.

4. Find meaning and purpose: Engaging in activities that give you a sense of meaning and purpose can help you stay motivated and maintain a positive outlook on life.

Conclusion:

Cultivating resilience, adaptability, and a positive attitude can help us thrive as we age. By practicing self-care, building a support network, staying curious, embracing change, and focusing on the present moment, we can develop the skills we need to face life's challenges with confidence and resilience.

7.2.3 - Embracing the wisdom and insights gained through life experiences

As we age, we accumulate a wealth of knowledge and experiences that shape who we are and how we view the world. Embracing this wisdom and using it to our advantage can have a positive impact on our well-being and overall aging experience. Here are some ways to embrace the wisdom and insights gained through life experiences:

1. Reflect on your past experiences: Take time to reflect on the challenges, triumphs, and lessons learned throughout your life. Consider how these experiences have shaped who you are today and how you can use this knowledge to navigate future challenges.

2. Share your stories: Share your stories with others, whether it's with friends, family, or in a community setting. By sharing your experiences, you not only pass down your wisdom but also build meaningful connections with others.

3. Mentor others: Consider becoming a mentor or volunteering in a role where you can use your experiences to guide and support others. Mentoring can be a mutually beneficial relationship, as you can also learn from the mentee and their experiences.

4. Embrace lifelong learning: Even with a lifetime of experiences, there is always something new to learn. Embrace a growth mindset and seek out opportunities to learn and expand your knowledge.

5. Stay curious: Curiosity is key to staying engaged and active as we age. Keep exploring new interests, hobbies, and experiences to stay mentally and physically stimulated.

By embracing the wisdom and insights gained through life experiences, we can not only enhance our own well-being but also make a positive impact on those around us.

7.2.4 - Harnessing the power of self-compassion and forgiveness

As we age, it is common to accumulate emotional baggage, regrets, and guilt from past experiences that can weigh us down and affect our overall well-being. Learning how to practice self-compassion and forgiveness can help us let go of these negative emotions and move forward towards a happier and healthier life.

Self-compassion is the act of treating ourselves with kindness and understanding, even in moments of difficulty and suffering. It involves acknowledging our pain and suffering without judgment or criticism, and extending the same level of care and support that we would offer to a close friend or loved one. By practicing self-compassion, we can cultivate a greater sense of self-worth, reduce feelings of shame and inadequacy, and develop a more positive outlook on life.

Forgiveness, on the other hand, is the act of letting go of resentment, anger, or blame towards ourselves or others. It does not mean forgetting or condoning harmful actions, but rather releasing the emotional burden associated with them and moving on with our lives. By practicing forgiveness, we can free ourselves from the negative effects of grudges and resentments, and promote emotional healing and growth.

Here are some practical tips for cultivating self-compassion and forgiveness in your life:

1. Practice mindfulness: Mindfulness is the act of being present and aware in the current moment, without judgment or distraction. By practicing mindfulness, we can become more attuned to our thoughts, feelings, and bodily sensations, and learn to respond to them with greater compassion and understanding.

2. Challenge your inner critic: We all have an inner critic that can be harsh and judgmental towards ourselves. By learning to challenge and reframe these negative thoughts, we can cultivate a greater sense of self-compassion and self-acceptance.

3. Practice gratitude: Focusing on the positive aspects of our lives and expressing gratitude for them can help us develop a more positive outlook and cultivate greater self-compassion.

4. Take responsibility for your actions: When we take responsibility for our actions and choices, we can learn from our mistakes and move forward with greater self-awareness and compassion.

5. Seek support: Talking to a trusted friend, family member, or therapist can help us process difficult emotions, gain new perspectives, and develop greater self-compassion and forgiveness.

By cultivating self-compassion and forgiveness, we can learn to let go of negative emotions, cultivate a greater sense of self-worth and acceptance, and live a more fulfilling and joyful life as we age.

7.3: Nurturing Meaningful Connections and Pursuing Passions

7.3.1 - Strengthening and expanding your social network for lasting fulfillment

Humans are social creatures, and social relationships are an essential aspect of human well-being. Strong social connections have been linked to better physical and mental health, increased happiness and life satisfaction, and even longevity. Therefore, it is crucial to cultivate and maintain positive social relationships throughout life, especially as we age.

As we get older, our social network tends to shrink as our friends and loved ones pass away or move away. This can lead to social isolation and loneliness, which can have negative effects on our health and well-being. However, it is never too late to start building new relationships and expanding our social network.

Here are some tips for strengthening and expanding your social network:

1. Join clubs or groups that interest you: Joining a club or group based on your interests can be a great way to meet like-minded people. Whether it's a book club, a hiking group, or a cooking

class, you'll have the opportunity to socialize with people who share your passions.

2. Volunteer: Volunteering can be an excellent way to meet new people while also giving back to your community. Whether you volunteer at a local food bank or animal shelter, you'll have the opportunity to connect with others who share your values and interests.

3. Attend community events: Attending community events such as festivals, farmers markets, or concerts can be a fun way to meet new people and connect with your community.

4. Take classes: Taking classes at a local community college or learning center can be a great way to meet new people and learn new skills. Whether it's a foreign language class, an art workshop, or a cooking class, you'll have the opportunity to connect with others while expanding your horizons.

5. Use technology: Social media platforms and online communities can be an excellent way to connect with others who share your interests. You can also use technology to stay in touch with family and friends who live far away.

6. Stay in touch with old friends: Don't forget about the friends and loved ones you've already made. Staying in touch with old friends and acquaintances can help you maintain strong social connections and even reconnect with people you may have lost touch with.

7. Be open to new experiences: Finally, be open to new experiences and opportunities. Saying yes to new invitations or trying new things can lead to new friendships and connections.

In conclusion, building and maintaining positive social relationships is an essential aspect of healthy aging. By following these tips and being open to new experiences and connections, you can strengthen and expand your social network for lasting fulfillment.

7.3.2 - Pursuing your passions and discovering new interests

As we age, it's important to stay engaged in activities that bring us joy and purpose. Pursuing our passions and discovering new interests can provide a sense of fulfillment and contribute to a more fulfilling life. In this chapter, we'll explore the benefits of pursuing our passions and discovering new interests and provide practical tips for incorporating them into our lives.

Benefits of Pursuing Your Passions and Discovering New Interests

1. Improved Mental Health: Pursuing our passions and discovering new interests can provide a sense of purpose and direction, reducing feelings of depression and anxiety.

2. Increased Social Connections: Pursuing our passions can connect us with like-minded individuals, providing opportunities for social connection and engagement.

3. Enhanced Brain Function: Engaging in mentally stimulating activities, such as learning a new language or playing an

instrument, can improve cognitive function and memory retention.

4. Reduced Stress: Engaging in activities we enjoy can provide a sense of relaxation and reduce stress levels.

5. Increased Sense of Fulfillment: Pursuing our passions and discovering new interests can provide a sense of fulfillment and purpose in life, contributing to overall happiness and well-being.

Tips for Incorporating New Passions and Interests into Your Life

1. Take Small Steps: Incorporating new passions and interests into your life can be overwhelming, so start small. Take a class, attend a workshop, or simply spend a few hours engaging in an activity you enjoy.

2. Try New Things: Don't be afraid to try new things. Be open to new experiences and be willing to step outside of your comfort zone.

3. Follow Your Curiosity: If you're not sure what your passions are, follow your curiosity. Take note of the activities and subjects that interest you and explore them further.

4. Make Time: It's important to make time for the things we enjoy. Schedule time for your passions and interests just as you would any other appointment.

5. Connect with Others: Join a club, take a class, or attend an event related to your passions and interests. Connecting with others who share your interests can provide a sense of community and support.

Incorporating new passions and interests into your life can provide a sense of purpose and fulfillment, contributing to overall well-being. Whether it's learning a new skill, trying a new hobby, or connecting with like-minded individuals, the benefits of pursuing our passions and discovering new interests are endless.

7.3.3 - Building a legacy of love, wisdom, and impact

As we age, we may start to think about what kind of legacy we want to leave behind. A legacy is more than just the material possessions we leave to our loved ones. It encompasses the impact we have had on the world, the wisdom we have gained and shared, and the love we have given and received.

Building a legacy is not just for the wealthy or famous. It is something that anyone can do, regardless of their financial or social status. In fact, building a legacy is often more about the intangible things that we leave behind rather than the tangible.

Here are some ways to build a legacy of love, wisdom, and impact:

1. Share your story and wisdom.

As we age, we gain a wealth of knowledge and experience. One way to leave a legacy is to share our stories and wisdom with those around us. We can do this by writing our memoirs, sharing stories with our loved ones, or volunteering to speak to younger generations about our experiences.

2. Give back to your community.

Another way to leave a lasting impact is to give back to your community. Whether it is volunteering at a local charity, donating to a cause you care about, or mentoring a young person, every small act of kindness can have a ripple effect that lasts far beyond our own lifetime.

3. Live a life of purpose.

Living a life of purpose means aligning our actions and choices with our values and beliefs. When we live a purposeful life, we leave a legacy of integrity and authenticity that can inspire others to do the same.

4. Love deeply and unconditionally.

Love is one of the most powerful legacies we can leave behind. By loving deeply and unconditionally, we create a ripple effect of kindness and compassion that can touch countless lives.

5. Embrace your creativity.

Creative expression is a unique way to leave a lasting legacy. Whether it is through writing, painting, music, or any other form of creative expression, we can leave behind something that speaks to the human experience and inspires others to embrace their own creativity.

In conclusion, building a legacy of love, wisdom, and impact is something that anyone can do, regardless of their age or background. By sharing our stories and wisdom, giving back to our communities, living a life of purpose, loving deeply, and embracing our creativity, we can leave a lasting legacy that will inspire and impact generations to come.

7.3.4 - The power of gratitude and living in the present moment

Gratitude is a powerful emotion that has been found to have numerous benefits for our mental and physical health. It is a practice of focusing on the positive aspects of life, appreciating what we have rather than what we lack. In this chapter, we will explore the science behind gratitude and its relationship with healthy aging. We will also discuss the benefits of living in the present moment and how it can enhance our well-being.

Gratitude and Healthy Aging

Studies have shown that gratitude is associated with better physical and mental health, improved sleep quality, reduced stress and depression, and increased resilience. In the context of aging, gratitude can help us maintain a positive outlook and cope with the challenges that come with age-related changes. It can also enhance our social connections and sense of purpose, which are important factors for healthy aging.

Research has shown that gratitude interventions, such as keeping a gratitude journal or writing letters of appreciation, can increase feelings of gratitude and improve well-being. A study published in the Journal of Personality and Social

Psychology found that participants who wrote letters expressing gratitude reported higher levels of happiness and life satisfaction, and lower levels of depression, compared to a control group.

Living in the Present Moment

Living in the present moment, also known as mindfulness, is another practice that has been found to have numerous benefits for our well-being. Mindfulness involves paying attention to our present moment experiences with openness, curiosity, and non-judgment. It can help us reduce stress and anxiety, improve our relationships, and enhance our cognitive and emotional functioning.

In the context of aging, mindfulness can help us cope with the challenges of aging and cultivate a sense of appreciation for the present moment. It can also help us develop a greater sense of self-awareness and acceptance, which can be beneficial for our mental and emotional well-being.

Research has shown that mindfulness interventions, such as meditation and yoga, can improve cognitive function, reduce stress and anxiety, and improve quality of life. A study published in the Journal of Alternative and Complementary Medicine found that participants who practiced mindfulness meditation had improved immune function and reduced inflammation compared to a control group.

Conclusion

Gratitude and mindfulness are powerful practices that can enhance our well-being and support healthy aging. By focusing on the positive aspects of our lives and cultivating a sense of appreciation for the present moment, we can improve our mental and physical health and build resilience to the challenges that come with aging. Incorporating gratitude and mindfulness practices into our daily lives can help us lead a more fulfilling and joyful life, regardless of our age.

7.4: The Ageless Odyssey Continues

7.4.1 - Celebrating your achievements and milestones on the journey to agelessness

As you embark on your journey towards agelessness, it is important to celebrate your achievements and milestones along the way. Aging is a process that can be filled with challenges and setbacks, but it is also a journey that can be marked with moments of triumph and success. By taking the time to acknowledge and celebrate these moments, you can build momentum and stay motivated on your path towards optimal well-being.

Here are some ways to celebrate your achievements and milestones on the journey to agelessness:

1. Reflect on Your Progress: Take some time to reflect on your progress so far. Think about the changes you have made and the milestones you have achieved. Celebrate the progress you have made and acknowledge the hard work and dedication that went into getting there.

2. Share Your Achievements with Others: Sharing your achievements with others can help you stay motivated and accountable. Tell your friends and family about your successes and how you achieved them. You may inspire others to embark on their own journey towards agelessness.

3. Treat Yourself: Treat yourself to something special when you reach a milestone. It could be something small like buying yourself a new book or taking a relaxing bath, or something bigger like planning a vacation or buying a piece of jewelry. Whatever it is, make sure it is something that makes you feel happy and accomplished.

4. Create a Memory: Create a memory to commemorate your achievement. Take a photo, make a scrapbook, or write in a journal. This will help you remember and celebrate your success for years to come.

5. Set New Goals: After you celebrate your achievements, set new goals to keep yourself moving forward. Use your accomplishments as motivation to continue on your journey towards agelessness.

Remember, celebrating your achievements and milestones is not only a way to acknowledge your progress but also to motivate and inspire you to continue on your path towards optimal well-being. By taking the time to celebrate your successes, you can build resilience and stay committed to living your best life at any age.

7.4.2 - Embracing the unknown and the potential for growth and transformation

As we age, we often face uncertainty and the unknown, which can be challenging to navigate. However, it is important to embrace the unknown as an opportunity for growth and transformation. In this chapter, we will explore the importance of embracing the unknown and how it can lead to a more fulfilling and satisfying life.

1. The Importance of Embracing the Unknown

One of the main challenges of aging is the uncertainty of the future. We may face health challenges, changes in our social networks, and other life transitions that can be difficult to navigate. However, embracing the unknown can be an opportunity for growth and transformation. Here are some reasons why:

- It can lead to personal growth: When we face the unknown, we have the opportunity to learn and grow. We can develop new skills, gain new insights, and discover new aspects of ourselves.

- It can increase resilience: Embracing the unknown can help us build resilience and adaptability. We can learn to cope with uncertainty and become more flexible in the face of change.

- It can lead to new opportunities: When we embrace the unknown, we open ourselves up to new possibilities and opportunities that we may not have considered before. This can lead to new experiences and a more fulfilling life.

2. Strategies for Embracing the Unknown

While embracing the unknown can be challenging, there are strategies we can use to help us navigate uncertainty and find growth and transformation. Here are some strategies to consider:

- Practice mindfulness: Mindfulness can help us stay present and focused, even in the face of uncertainty. By cultivating mindfulness, we can develop a greater sense of calm and acceptance in the face of the unknown.

- Cultivate a growth mindset: A growth mindset involves viewing challenges and setbacks as opportunities for growth and learning. By adopting a growth mindset, we can approach the unknown with a sense of curiosity and openness.

- Take small steps: When facing the unknown, it can be helpful to take small steps and break things down into manageable pieces. This can help us avoid feeling overwhelmed and stay focused on our goals.

- Seek support: It is important to seek support when facing uncertainty. This can include seeking advice from friends and family, consulting with a therapist, or joining a support group.

3. Conclusion

Embracing the unknown can be challenging, but it can also be an opportunity for growth and transformation. By cultivating mindfulness, adopting a growth mindset, taking small steps, and seeking support, we can navigate uncertainty with greater ease and find fulfillment and satisfaction in our lives.

7.4.3 - The ongoing evolution of longevity research and innovation

Introduction

The field of longevity research and innovation has been rapidly growing in recent years, with many breakthroughs and advancements in our understanding of the aging process and how it can be slowed, halted, or even reversed. This chapter will explore some of the most exciting developments in longevity research and innovation, including recent breakthroughs, ongoing studies, and emerging trends.

Recent Breakthroughs in Longevity Research

In recent years, there have been many exciting breakthroughs in the field of longevity research, including:

1. Cellular Reprogramming: Cellular reprogramming is a technique that involves changing one type of cell into another type of cell, such as changing a skin cell into a neuron. This technique has shown promise in reversing age-related damage to cells and tissues, and may eventually be used to reverse the aging process itself.

2. Senolytics: Senolytics are drugs that target and eliminate senescent cells, which are cells that have stopped dividing and are no longer functioning properly. Senescent cells are thought to contribute to the aging process, and eliminating them may help to slow or even reverse the aging process.

3. NAD+ Boosters: NAD+ boosters are supplements that increase the levels of NAD+ in the body. NAD+ is a molecule that plays a key role in energy production, DNA repair, and other cellular processes that are important for maintaining health and longevity. By boosting NAD+ levels, these supplements may help to promote healthy aging.

4. Gene Editing: Gene editing is a technique that involves making changes to DNA, such as repairing or replacing damaged genes. This technique has shown promise in treating genetic diseases and may eventually be used to extend lifespan and promote healthy aging.

Ongoing Studies in Longevity Research

There are many ongoing studies in the field of longevity research, including:

1. The TAME Study: The TAME (Targeting Aging with Metformin) study is a clinical trial that is testing the effectiveness of the drug metformin in delaying or preventing age-related diseases. The study aims to show that targeting aging itself, rather than individual diseases, is a viable approach to improving healthspan and lifespan.

2. The Longevity Consortium: The Longevity Consortium is a collaborative effort between researchers, clinicians, and industry partners to advance our understanding of aging and develop new interventions to promote healthy aging. The consortium is focused on identifying the genetic, environmental, and lifestyle factors that contribute to aging, and developing new therapies to target these factors.

3. The National Institute on Aging Interventions Testing Program: The National Institute on Aging Interventions Testing Program is a program that tests potential anti-aging interventions in mice to determine their effectiveness in promoting healthy aging. The program has identified several promising interventions, including rapamycin and acarbose, which are now being tested in clinical trials.

Emerging Trends in Longevity Research

There are several emerging trends in the field of longevity research, including:

1. AI and Machine Learning: AI and machine learning are being used to analyze large datasets and identify patterns and relationships that may be difficult or impossible for humans to detect. This technology may help researchers to better understand the complex biological processes that contribute to aging and identify new targets for intervention.

2. Personalized Medicine: Personalized medicine involves tailoring medical treatments to the individual patient based on their genetic, environmental, and lifestyle factors. This approach may be particularly effective in promoting healthy aging, as it allows for targeted interventions that are tailored to the unique needs of each individual.

3. Nutrigenomics: Nutrigenomics is the study of how the foods we eat affect our genes and how this affects our health and aging. This field is rapidly growing, and may

7.4.4 - Staying informed and adapting to new discoveries and technologies in the field of aging

As we continue to explore the possibilities of living longer, healthier lives, it is important to stay informed about the latest discoveries and technologies in the field of aging. In order to maintain optimal health and well-being as we age, we must be willing to adapt to new ideas and embrace change. This chapter will explore the importance of staying informed and adapting to new discoveries and technologies in the field of aging.

One of the key ways to stay informed about new developments in the field of aging is to stay up-to-date with the latest research. Advances in genetics, epigenetics, and other areas of science are providing new insights into the aging process, and it is important to keep abreast of these discoveries. This can involve reading scientific journals, attending conferences and seminars, and following experts in the field on social media.

Another important way to stay informed is to stay connected with others who are interested in aging research and innovation. This can involve joining online communities, attending meetups, and participating in forums and discussions. By connecting with others who share our interests, we can learn from their experiences and gain new insights into the latest developments in the field.

Adapting to new discoveries and technologies in the field of aging is also crucial for maintaining optimal health and well-being as we age. For example, new technologies such as wearable health monitors and digital health platforms can help us monitor our health and make informed decisions about our lifestyle and medical care. Genetic testing can also provide valuable information about our risk for certain diseases and conditions, allowing us to take proactive steps to prevent or manage them.

In addition, emerging research is revealing new ways to enhance our health and well-being as we age. For example, studies have shown that regular exercise, a healthy diet, and adequate sleep can all have significant benefits for our physical and mental health as we age. Mindfulness practices such as meditation and yoga can also be effective tools for managing stress and promoting well-being.

Finally, staying informed and adapting to new discoveries and technologies in the field of aging can help us maintain a sense of purpose and meaning as we age. By continuing to learn and grow, we can remain engaged in our communities and contribute to the world around us. Whether through volunteering, mentoring, or pursuing new interests, we can continue to make a positive impact on the world as we age.

In conclusion, staying informed and adapting to new discoveries and technologies in the field of aging is crucial for maintaining optimal health and well-being as we age. By staying connected with others who share our interests, keeping abreast of the latest research, and embracing new ideas and technologies, we can continue to thrive and make meaningful contributions to the world around us.

Ending

the journey to agelessness is a rich and fulfilling odyssey that encompasses every aspect of our lives. This book has provided you with a comprehensive roadmap, delving into the many dimensions of longevity, from the cellular mechanisms that govern the aging process to the lifestyle choices, mental resilience, self-care practices, and social connections that contribute to a vibrant and healthy life.

We have also explored the power of technology and scientific innovation in shaping the future of aging, including the role of digital health, wearable technologies, virtual and augmented reality, robotics, and personalized genomics. As we forge ahead into the uncharted territory of our own ageless odyssey, it is essential to stay informed and adapt to new discoveries and advances in the field of aging.

Throughout the chapters, we have underscored the importance of personalizing your approach to longevity and well-being. By assessing your unique needs, goals, and circumstances, you can create a tailored plan that integrates the strategies and insights gleaned from the various aspects of this book. Equally important is cultivating a resilient mindset, embracing the wisdom and insights gained from life experiences, and nurturing meaningful connections with others.

The journey to agelessness is not a destination, but a continuous process of growth, exploration, and adaptation. As you embark on this odyssey, remember to celebrate your achievements and milestones along the way, revel in the present moment, and express gratitude for the opportunity to live a vibrant, healthy, and fulfilling life.

Embrace the unknown, harness the power of transformation, and stay committed to your ageless journey. Ultimately, the key to longevity lies not in mere physical survival, but in living a life filled with passion, purpose, and joy, surrounded by loved ones, and contributing positively to the world around us. By doing so, we can transcend the limits of age and truly embrace the ageless odyssey that awaits us.